CARDIOPULMONARY CEREBRAL RESUSCITATION

by

Peter Safar

Prepared for the World Federation of Societies of Anaesthesiologists.

Written for physicians of all disciplines, nurses and paramedical personnel, to enhance their ability to resuscitate; and for physician and non-physician resuscitation instructors and organizers. Parts of Chapters I and V are also suitable for non-medical personnel.

A color slide set of illustrations in this book is available from the distributors.

Published and printed by Asmund S. Laerdal, Stavanger, Norway, 1981.
Available through bookstores worldwide by W.B. Saunders Co., Philadelphia — Toronto — London.
Available in bulk to institutions through the WFSA's appointed representatives
— for USA, Canada, UK: W.B. Saunders Co., Philadelphia — Toronto — London, respectively.
— for other countries: Asmund S. Laerdal, P.O. Box 377, N4001 Stavanger, Norway.

ISBN 82 - 990738 - 0 - 4

To
the memory of
ELIZABETH and HANNI
and others
who needed and taught
resuscitation
and love

FOREWORD

One of the most important goals of the World Federation of Societies of Anaesthesiologists (WFSA) is the progress of the methods of resuscitation throughout the world. For this reason the Committee on Cardio-Pulmonary Resuscitation (CPR) of the World Federation of Societies of Anaesthesiologists in 1965 asked a world pioneer of resuscitation, Peter Safar, Professor of Anaesthesiology at the University of Pittsburgh, Pennsylvania, to write a manual on CPR.

A generous grant from the Asmund Laerdal Company, which also printed the manual, led to its worldwide distribution starting with the WFSA Congress in London in September 1968. Between 1968 and 1978 about 250,000 copies were distributed gratis or sold at cost throughout the world. These copies were printed in 15 languages.

At the WFSA meeting in Kyoto in 1972 the manual was praised as a major contribution of WFSA, and Peter Safar deserves great credit for its success.

The impact of the simplicity of modern CPR as presented in the manual's first edition is retained in the second edition, but the need for many advances beyond basic life support, particularly the logical expansion of CPR to Cardiopulmonary-Cerebral Resuscitation (CPCR) has necessitated an entirely new manual for the 1980's.

In the second edition the author, Peter Safar, has synthesized accepted and proven techniques, his own clinical teaching and research experiences in resuscitation over 30 years, together with new concepts and possibilities.

Anaesthesiologists have pioneered much of the initiating research, training mechanisms and delivery programs of CPR since the 1950's. CPCR, which represents the acute phase of critical care medicine (intensive therapy), should, however, be pursued with multidisciplinary participation and contribution.

It is hoped that anaesthesiologists will retain and expand their roles as initiators, teachers, leaders and team members in resuscitation around the world.

by Rudolf Frey
Dr.med., F.F.A.R.C.S.
Mainz 1981

Chairman of the Committee
on Cardio-Pulmonary
Resuscitation of the
World Federation of Societies
of Anaesthesiologists

Professor of Anaesthesiology
Johannes Gutenberg-University
D-6500 Mainz
F.R. Germany

4

PREFACE

The first modern resuscitation manuals written in the 1950's were on rescue breathing, and those written in the 1960's on cardiopulmonary resuscitation. The latter included a 48-page manual solicited by the World Federation of Societies of Anaesthesiologists' (WFSA) Cardiopulmonary Resuscitation (CPR) Committee. The present second edition is actually a new book, as it represents an attempt to meet the demand for more sophisticated knowledge, increased opportunities for reversing dying processes, increasingly complex methods, and the expansion of CPR to cardiopulmonary-cerebral resuscitation (CPCR). Since good patient outcome often depends not only on the speed and quality of emergency resuscitation, but also on long-term resuscitation (intensive care) — which includes support of recovery of the target organ, the brain — the author has included a brief review of recommended measures for post-resuscitative life support.

The objective of this manual is to convey the *knowledge* which should be acquired prior to skill practice, resuscitation attempts on patients, and the organization and conduct of training programs in basic and advanced life support. A manual cannot teach vital *skills*, which can only be acquired through practice — on mannequins, on other trainees and on patients.

This manual is for physicians and paramedical instructors of cardiopulmonary resuscitation, basic and advanced life support. Some colleagues will disagree with some of the knowledge items taught. It is impossible to obtain an international or even national consensus on *what* to teach *whom* and *how*, since this field is dynamic.

However, CPR *guidelines* (recommendations) have been developed by national and international groups since the 1960's. Regarding the question of what to teach to nonmedical personnel, it is important that the materials be kept simple and uniform within each country, to avoid confusion and hesitation in performance in the situation of an actual case. For basic life support by lay persons, international guidelines are desirable and feasible. Medical personnel, however, should have general flexible guidelines which do not hinder innovations. *Standards* imply that they are rigidly based on hard data, which usually is not possible in medicine, and suggest punitive action for noncompliance, which is inappropriate and distasteful. Thus, we prefer to talk of «guidelines» which are sufficiently flexible to permit change when solid documentation of the life saving or the teaching advantages of new techniques have been provided.

This manual reflects majority agreement by the members of the World Federation of Societies of Anaesthesiologists' CPR Committee. Most of the techniques taught in this manual had been incorporated into recommendations by the American Heart Association, National Research Council (U.S.A.) and several countries' national and international Red Cross societies. It is important that medical personnel maintain sufficient flexibility regarding guidelines to take into account the differing resources, priorities and cultural constraints in various countries around the globe. Thus, resuscitation leaders in each country should feel free to modify the contents of this manual, if this improves acceptability and implementation of resuscitation services in their environment.

The science «resuscitology» and the care delivery mechanisms «emergency and critical care medicine» (intensive therapy) are multidisciplinary endeavors. While some anesthesiologists were initiators of modern resuscitation, their present involvement as researchers, clinical leaders, team members, consultants or teachers will depend on personal interest, availability and competence, and on local circumstances. We hope that this manual will help all types of professionals to skillfully reverse, either personally or indirectly, acute dying processes in patients whose time to die has not yet come. The goal, of course, is restoration of new life with quality, including human mentation.

Peter Safar
Pittsburgh, 1981

ACKNOWLEDGEMENTS

For the ability and opportunity to contribute, I am grateful to my parents, teachers, colleagues and friends, and the University of Pittsburgh. For maintaining the home, while tolerating a workaholic, I thank my wife Eva and my sons Philip and Paul. For help with completion of the manuscript, thanks go to the staff of the Resuscitation Research Center, University of Pittsburgh (Nancy Moran, Tancy Crawford, Carmela Falchetti); to H. Eikeland; to the World Federation of Societies of Anaesthesiologists' Committee on Cardiopulmonary Resuscitation and Critical Care (Doctors R. Frey, Germany; Tess Brophy, Australia; Nancy Caroline, Israel; E. Hulsz, Mexico; Z. Vieira, Brazil; J. Zorab, Britain); and to Doctors N. Abramson, P. Baskett, P. Berkebile, N. Bircher, A. Grenvik, J. Lane, B. Lind, and J. Redding. Doctors Caroline, Zorab and Baskett provided valuable editorial help.

Special credit goes to Asmund Laerdal, who has supported resuscitation for two decades as inventor, designer, manufacturer and patron of cardiopulmonary resuscitation teaching materials, symposia and guidelines.

Peter Safar
Pittsburgh 1981

CONTENTS

Introduction and History 10
Phases and Steps of CPCR *(Fig. 1, Tbl. I)* 11

PHASE ONE BASIC LIFE SUPPORT
Emergency Oxygenation

Chapter I A

Airway Control

Causes of Airway Obstruction 16
Recognition of Airway Obstruction 17
Emergency Airway Control Measures *(Tbl. I)* 17
Backward Tilt of Head *(Fig. 2)*. 18
Positioning *(Fig. 3)* 19
Positive Pressure Inflation Attempts *(Fig. 4)*. 21
Triple Airway Maneuver (Head Tilt, Mouth Open, Jaw Thrust) *(Fig. 5)* 21
Manual Clearing of the Airway *(Fig. 6)* 24
Blows and Thrusts for Foreign Body Obstruction *(Fig. 7, 8, 9)*. 25
Clearing the Airway by Suction *(Fig. 10)*. 29
Pharyngeal Intubation *(Fig. 11)*. 30
Esophageal Obturator Airway Insertion *(Fig. 12)*. 32
Tracheal Intubation *(Fig. 13, 14, 15, Tbl.II)*. 35
Alternatives to Tracheal Intubation. 48
–Cricothyrotomy *(Fig. 16)*. 49
–Translaryngeal Jet Insufflation *(Fig. 17)* 50
Other Steps of Airway Control. 51
– Tracheotomy *(Fig. 18)*. 51
– Bronchoscopy, Bronchodilation, Pleural Drainage *(Fig. 19)*. 53

Chapter I B

Breathing Support *(Emergency Artificial Ventilation and Oxygenation)*

Ventilation Patterns *(Fig. 20)* 56
Direct Mouth-to-Mouth and Mouth-to-Nose Ventilation *(Fig. 21)*. 58
Mouth-to-Adjunct Ventilation 61
– Mouth-to-Airway 62
– Mouth-to-Mask with Oxygen *(Fig. 22)* 62
Bag-Valve-Mask with Oxygen *(Fig. 23)* 64
Manually-Triggered Oxygen-Powered Ventilators. 67
Automatic Ventilators 68
Oxygen Delivery Systems *(Fig. 24)*. 70
Selecting Ventilation and Oxygenation Techniques *(Tbl.III)* 72

Chapter I C

Circulation Support *(Cardiac Resuscitation)*

Causes of Cardiac Arrest. 76
Recognition of Cardiac Arrest *(Fig. 25)*. 76
Closed Chest Cardiopulmonary Resuscitation *(Fig. 26, 27)* 77
Combinations of Ventilation and Sternal Compressions *(Fig. 28, 29)*. 81
Control of Hemorrhage *(Fig. 30, 31)* 87
Extrication and Positioning for Shock *(Fig. 32)*. 91

PHASE TWO **ADVANCED LIFE SUPPORT**
Restoration of Spontaneous Circulation

Chapter II

Drugs and Fluids

Routes for Drugs and Fluids 94
−Peripheral Intravenous Route *(Fig. 33)*. 94
−Intrapulmonary Route. 95
− Intracardiac Route 97
− Intramuscular Route 98
− Central Venous Route 98
− Pulmonary Artery Catheterization 99
− Arterial Puncture and Catheterization *(Fig. 34)* 100
Drugs *(Fig. 35)*. 102
Fluids 116

Electrocardiographic Diagnosis

Techniques of Electrocardiography. 121
EKG Patterns of Cardiac Arrest *(Fig. 36)* 123
Life-Threatening Dysrhythmias *(Fig. 37, 38, 39)*. 124

Fibrillation Treatment (Defibrillation) *(Fig. 40, 41)* 131

PHASE THREE **PROLONGED LIFE SUPPORT**
Post-Resuscitative Brain-Oriented Therapy

Chapter III

Intensive Therapy with Cerebral Resuscitation

Respiratory and Cardiovascular Support *(Tbl. IV)*. 138
Standard Measures of Brain-oriented Life Support *(Tbl. V)*. 140
Special Measures for Brain Resuscitation *(Tbl. VI)*. 144

Evaluation and Critical Care Triage

Definitions of Death 148
Evaluation ("Gauging") 149
Evaluation of Insult, Coma, Outcome *(Tbl. VII, VIII)* 149
When Not to Undertake Emergency Resuscitation..................153
When to Terminate Emergency Resuscitation.....................153
When to Terminate Long-term Resuscitation *(Tbl. IX)*...............155
How to Terminate Long-term Resuscitation in total Brain Death *(Tbl. X)* ..155
How to Terminate Long-term Resuscitation in Vegetative State *(Tbl. IX)*...160

Chapter IV

Special Considerations

Resuscitation of Infants and Children *(Fig. 42, Tbl. XI)*..............161
Witnessed Sudden Cardiac Death *(Fig. 43)*......................169
Open Chest Cardiopulmonary Resuscitation *(Fig. 44)* 172
Cardiac Arrest due to Exsanguination 174
Near-Drowning...177
Myocardial Ischemia and Infarction. Sudden Cardiac Death 178
Miscellaneous Conditions requiring Resuscitation 180
Complications and Pitfalls of CPR 181

Chapter V

Teaching of First Aid and Resuscitation

What to Teach to Whom *(Tbl. XII)*............................183
Teaching the Lay Public....................................186
Teaching Health Care Personnel...............................188
Teaching Methodology *(Fig. 45, Tbl. XIII)*.....................189
Testing *(Tbl. XIV - XVIII)* 198

Chapter VI

Organization

Hospital-wide Organization 204
Community-wide Organization *(Tbl. XIX)*.......................206
Advanced Life Support Units.................................210
Legal Considerations 214
Conclusions 215
Glossary (Abbreviations, Definitions, Normal Values) 217
Bibliography..220
Index 231
Case Report Form.......................................239

INTRODUCTION AND HISTORY

Potentially reversible airway obstruction, hypoventilation, apnea, blood loss, pulselessness (cardiac arrest) and brain injury are among the leading causes of death resulting from accidents, heart attacks and other medical emergencies. The leading causes of preventable sudden death before old age are ventricular fibrillation (in patients over age 44) from asymptomatic ischemic heart disease; nontraumatic accidents (e.g., drowning, poisoning); and trauma (in patients under age 38) caused by the violence of man or accidents.

Irreversible brain damage may occur when cessation of circulation (cardiac arrest) lasts longer than a few minutes (the precise time limits being currently under reinvestigation); or after trauma, when severe hypoxemia or blood loss remain uncorrected. However, the immediate application of modern resuscitation is often capable of preventing biologic death. Resuscitative measures can be initiated anywhere without the use of equipment, by trained individuals, ranging from the lay public to physician specialists.

There were few immediately applicable effective emergency resuscitation techniques available before the 1950's, when modern respiratory resuscitation was pioneered; modern circulatory resuscitation began in the 1960's, and therapeutically promising research on brain resuscitation began in 1970. The latter work has extended cardiopulmonary resuscitation (CPR) to cardiopulmonary-cerebral resuscitation (CPCR). Resuscitation from circulatory shock has a longer history than that from cardiac arrest (Blalock). Intensive care (long-term resuscitation), essential for optimal outcome after emergency resuscitation, was initiated in Scandinavia and Baltimore in the 1950's and pioneered by several groups around the world in the 1960's (Nilsson, Ibsen, Safar, Holmdahl).

The development of modern CPR has been based largely on ideas conceived or accidentally discovered many years ago, which were rediscovered and re-explored since the 1950's. These include intermittent positive pressure artificial ventilation (IPPV) (Vesalius, 1543); mouth-to- mouth breathing (Tossach, 1771); jaw-thrust (Esmarch, 1878; Heiberg, 1874); open chest cardiac resuscitation (Boehm, 1878; Schiff, 1882); internal defibrillation (Prevost, 1899; Wiggers, 1940); tracheal intubation (Kuhn, 1911; Macintosh, 1920); external CPR (Maass, 1892); external defibrillation with direct current (Gurvitch, 1946); and pathophysiologic research on dying and resuscitation (Negovsky).

The history of modern CPR can be summarized according to a series of landmark developments during the past 25 to 30 years: Proof that ventilation with the operator's exhaled air is physiologically sound (Elam, 1954); proof of the ventilatory superiority of exhaled air ventilation (without equipment) over manual chest-pressure arm-lift maneuvers (Safar, 1958); studies showing why soft-tissue obstruction of the upper airway in unconscious patients could be prevented or corrected by backward tilt of the head, forward displacement of the mandible, and opening of the mouth (Safar, 1958); proof of the ventilatory superiority of exhaled air ventilation over chest pressure methods in children (Gordon, 1958); rediscovery and development of external cardiac compression (Kouwenhoven, 1960); demonstration of the need to combine positive pressure ventilation with external cardiac compression (Safar, 1961); intrathoracic electric defibrillation of the heart in human patients (Beck, 1947); the concept of «the heart too good to die» (Beck, 1960); external electric defibrillation of the heart in human patients (Zoll, 1956); electric cardiac pacing (Zoll, 1956); proof of the feasibility of teaching CPR to the lay public (Safar, 1958; Elam 1961; Lind, 1961; Winchell, 1966; Berkebile, 1973); proof that lay people in the field will perform mouth-to-mouth breathing (Elam, 1961; Lind, 1963) and CPR (Lund, 1976); production of realistic training aids by Laerdal since 1960; and agreements on details of techniques and teaching methods through many national committees and the international symposia of Stavanger (1961) (Poulsen) and Oslo (1967) (Lund), Norway.

Thus, over the past 30 years, old techniques have been refashioned into new systems. CPR works, and thousands of lives could be saved each year if enough individuals were properly trained in resuscitation. Clinical results depend heavily, however, upon perfection and uniformity of training and appropriate stress given to the importance of initiating resuscitation techniques at the earliest possible moment.

PHASES AND STEPS OF CARDIOPULMONARY-CEREBRAL RESUSCITATION (CPCR) (Tbl. I, Fig. 1)

For didactic purposes, we have divided CPCR into three phases: (I) Basic Life Support; (II) Advanced Life Support; (III) Prolonged Life Support; and into nine steps, using the letters of the alphabet from (A) through (I) (Tbl. I, Fig. 1).*

Phase I, basic life support, is for emergency oxygenation and consists of Steps *(A) Airway control; (B) Breathing support,* i.e., emergency artificial ventilation and oxygenation of the lungs; and *(C) Circulation support,* i.e., recognition of pulselessness and establishment of artificial circulation by cardiac compressions, control of hemorrhage, and positioning for shock.

As soon as feasible after initiation of Phase I, call for help, without interrupting CPR, and activate the community's Emergency Medical Services' (EMS) system (or the hospital CPR team response). Ask your helper to call the emergency number for an ambulance. Make sure you know this number. Say it is a resuscitation case. If you are alone, use your best judgment when to call, with minimal interruption of CPR. If no phone is available, continue CPR for at least one hour (if you consider him salvable) or until medical personnel can take over.

Phase II, advanced life support, is for restarting spontaneous circulation and stabilizing the cardiopulmonary system, by restoring near-normal arterial oxygen transport (i.e., arterial oxygen content times blood flow). Phase II consists of Steps *(D) Drugs and fluids* via intravenous infusion; *(E) Electrocardioscopy* (cardiography); and *(F) Fibrillation treatment,* usually by electric countershock.

The sequential actions in performing Phases I and II, which lead to the establishment of adequate spontaneous circulation, should be as rapid as possible, since artifical circulation by external (closed chest) cardiac compressions produces only 6 to 30 percent of normal blood flow. Open chest cardiac compressions are more effective and may produce 50 percent of normal blood flow; they cannot be used outside the hospital.

* Since the introduction of CPR, this author has used the term «basic life support» for Steps A, B, and C and «advanced life support» for Steps D, E and F, irrespective of the use of equipment. The American Heart Association on the other hand, uses the term «basic life support» for Steps A, B, and C without the use of equipment; and the term «advanced life support» for Steps A, B, and C with the use of equipment, plus Steps D through I.

Phase III, prolonged life support, is for postresuscitative intensive care. It consists of *(G) Gauging,* i.e., determining and treating the cause of death and assessing the patient's salvability; *(H) Human mentation* — to be restored hopefully by new brain resuscitation measures; and *(I) Intensive care* (long-term resuscitation). This phase represents brain-oriented intensive care for multiple organ failure in the post-resuscitative period.

Phase III, which deserves more attention than it has received in the past, should be continued until the patient regains consciousness, brain death has been certified, or his underlying disease makes further resuscitation efforts senseless.

Life supporting first aid comprises basic measures, without the use of equipment, to be learned by the general public. They include selected basic components of CPR Steps A (head-tilt, open mouth, jaw thrust) and B (direct mouth-to-mouth and mouth-to-nose ventilation); they do not include external cardiac compressions (ECC). Beyond CPR, life supporting first aid includes control of external hemorrhage (by manual compression, elevation and pressure bandage); rescue pull (extrication of the victim from a wreck); and positioning to maintain open airway, combat shock and prevent further injury.

Trauma-oriented CPCR utilizes the phases and steps of CPCR, but with several differences in emphasis: For Step (A), jawthrust and open mouth with moderate backward tilt of the head is favored over maximal backward tilt of the head, because of possible cervical spine injury by excessive manipulation of the neck. Head injury poses special indications and contra-indications for airway control techniques, as coughing and straining must be avoided. Chest injury requires one to consider the constant risk of tension pneumothorax. For Step (B), in the trauma-oriented approach, oxygenation is more often needed than artificial ventilation, since apnea is rare in trauma, while hypoxemia is common. For Step (C), control of hemorrhage is more often needed than chest compressions. For (D), fluid resuscitation, central venous life-line and other measures for treating traumatic shock are crucial and far more important than drugs. Steps (E) and (F) must be available for trauma cases, but are rarely needed except for cases of chest injury. Phase III is of paramount importance, particularly for multi-trauma with head-chest injury.

The phases and steps of CPCR are set out in Table I and Figure 1.

For target audiences, see Chapter V.

TABLE I

Phases, Steps, and Measures of Cardiopulmonary-Cerebral Resuscitation

Phases	Steps	Measures performed	

Establish unresponsiveness — Activate EMS system

Phases	Steps	WITHOUT equipment	WITH equipment
I BASIC LIFE SUPPORT – BLS (Emergency oxygenation)	**A**irway Control	(1) *Backward tilt of head *Supine aligned position *Stable side position (2) *Lung inflation attempts (3) *Triple airway maneuver (Jaw thrust, open mouth) (4) *Manual clearing of mouth and throat Back blows - manual thrusts	(5) Pharyngeal suctioning (6) Pharyngeal intubation (7) Esophageal obturator airway insertion (8) Endotracheal intubation Tracheobronchial suctioning (9) Cricothyrotomy Translaryngeal O$_2$ jet insufflation (10) Tracheotomy Bronchoscopy Bronchodilation Pleural drainage
	Breathing Support	*Mouth-to-mouth (nose) ventilation	Mouth-to-adjunct with or without O$_2$ Manual bag-mask (tube) ventilation with or without O$_2$ Hand-triggered O$_2$ ventilation Mechanical ventilation
	Circulation Support	*Control of ext. hemorrh. *Position for shock Pulse checking Manual chest compressions	Mechanical chest compressions Open chest direct cardiac compressions Pressure pants (MAST) for shock
II ADVANCED LIFE SUPPORT – ALS (Restoration of spontaneous circulation)	**D**rugs and Fluids		IV Lifeline
	Electrocardiography		EKG monitoring
	Fibrillation Treatment		Defibrillation
III PROLONGED LIFE SUPPORT – PLS (Cerebral resuscitation and post-resuscitation Intensive therapy)	**G**auging		Determine and treat cause of demise Determine salvageability
	Human mentation		Cerebral resuscitation
	Intensive care		Multiple organ support

*Life Supporting First Aid

CARDIOPULMONARY – CEREBRAL RESUSCITATION

PHASE ONE **BASIC LIFE SUPPORT**
Emergency Oxygenation

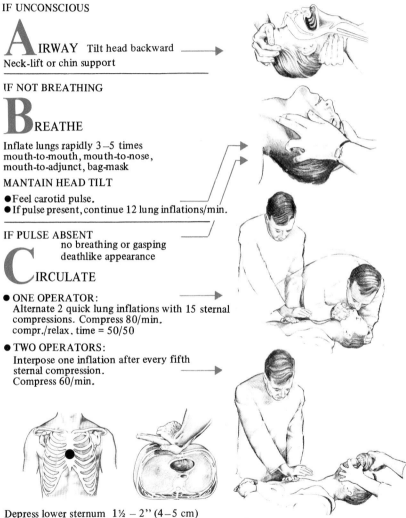

IF UNCONSCIOUS

A IRWAY Tilt head backward ⟶
Neck-lift or chin support

IF NOT BREATHING

B REATHE

Inflate lungs rapidly 3–5 times
mouth-to-mouth, mouth-to-nose,
mouth-to-adjunct, bag-mask

MANTAIN HEAD TILT

● Feel carotid pulse.
● If pulse present, continue 12 lung inflations/min.

IF PULSE ABSENT no breathing or gasping
deathlike appearance

C IRCULATE

● ONE OPERATOR:
Alternate 2 quick lung inflations with 15 sternal
compressions. Compress 80/min.
compr./relax. time = 50/50

● TWO OPERATORS:
Interpose one inflation after every fifth
sternal compression.
Compress 60/min.

Depress lower sternum 1½ – 2" (4–5 cm)
CONTINUE RESUSCITATION until spontaneous pulse returns

Figure 1 Phases and steps of cardiopulmonary – cerebral resuscitation

14

PHASE TWO **ADVANCED LIFE SUPPORT**
Restoration of Spontaneous Circulation

DO NOT INTERRUPT CARDIAC COMPRESSIONS AND LUNG VENTILATION
INTUBATE TRACHEA WHEN POSSIBLE

DRUGS AND FLUIDS, I.V. LIFELINE

EPINEPHRINE (ADRENALINE)
0.5 - 1.0 mg I.V. repeat larger dose as necessary

SODIUM BICARBONATE
1 mEq/kg I.V. if arrest over 2 min
Repeat dose every 10 minutes until pulse returns.
Monitor and normalize arterial pH

I.V. FLUIDS as indicated

E.K.G. Ventricular fibrillation ? Asystole ? Bizarre complexes ?

FIBRILLATION TREATMENT

EXTERNAL DEFIBRILLATION
D.C. 100 – 400 W sec. (Joules)
Repeat shock as necessary

LIDOCAINE (LIGNOCAINE)
1 – 2 mg/kg I.V. if necessary
continue I.V. infusion

IF ASYSTOLE
repeat D. Calcium and vasopressors as needed

CONTINUE RESUSCITATION until good pulse.
Restore normotension promptly

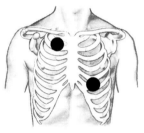

D.C. 100 – 400 W sec.

PHASE THREE **PROLONGED LIFE SUPPORT**
Post-Resuscitative Brain-Oriented Therapy

GAUGING Determine and treat cause of demise
Determine salvageability

HUMAN MENTATION - - CEREBRAL RESUSCITATION

INTENSIVE CARE

Immediately after restoration of spontaneous circulation and throughout coma - -
Ameliorate post-anoxic encephalopathy:
Monitoring (CV, art, (PA), bladder catheters; EKG)
Normotension. Oxygenation. Controlled Ventilation. Blood Variables. Temperature.
Relaxation. Anesthesia. Fluids. Electrolytes. Glucose. Alimentation. Drugs. (ICP).
(For Innovative Therapy see Chapter III)

BASIC LIFE SUPPORT
Emergency Oxygenation

Chapter I A

AIRWAY CONTROL

Causes of Airway Obstruction

The most common site of airway obstruction is hypopharyngeal (Fig. 2A), occurring in comatose patients when the relaxed tongue and neck muscles fail to lift the base of the tongue from the posterior pharyngeal wall, when the patient's head is in the flexed or mid-position. Holding the head tilted backward is therefore the most important first measure in resuscitation, since this maneuver stretches the anterior neck structures and thereby lifts the base of the tongue from the posterior pharyngeal wall (Safar). Sometimes additional forward displacement of the mandible (Esmarch, Heiberg) is required to produce this stretch, particularly when nasal obstruction necessitates opening of the mouth, which in turn reduces the stretch on anterior neck structures. The combination of the backward tilt of the head, forward displacement of the mandible and opening of the mouth constitutes the «triple airway maneuver» (Safar). In about one-third of unconscious patients the nasal passage is obstructed during exhalation because of valvelike behavior of the soft palate; moreover, the nose may be blocked by congestion, blood or mucus (Safar). When the chin is sagging, inspiratory efforts may «suck» the base of the tongue into an obstructing position (Guildner). Airway obstruction by the base of the tongue depends upon position of the head and jaw and can occur regardless of whether the patient is lateral, supine or prone (Safar, Asmussen). Although gravity may aid in the drainage of liquid foreign matter, it does not relieve hypopharyngeal soft tissue obstruction, and maneuvers to lift the base of the tongue, as described above, are required.

Another cause of airway obstruction is the presence in the upper airway of foreign matter such as vomitus or blood, which the unconscious patient cannot eliminate by swallowing or coughing. Laryngospasm is usually caused by upper airway stimulation in the stuporose or lightly comatose patient. Lower airway obstruction may be the result of bronchospasm, bronchial secretions, mucosal edema, inhaled gastric contents, or foreign matter.

Airway obstruction may be complete or partial. Complete obstruction is silent and leads to asphyxia (hypoxemia plus hypercarbia), apnea, and cardiac arrest (if not corrected) within 5 to 10 minutes. Partial obstruction is noisy and must also be promptly corrected, as it can result in hypoxic brain damage, cerebral or pulmonary edema or other complications; and may lead to exhaustion, secondary apnea and cardiac arrest.

Recognition of Airway Obstruction
Complete airway obstruction is recognized when one cannot hear or feel air flow at the mouth or nose. When there are spontaneous breathing movements, the presence of inspiratory retraction of supraclavicular and intercostal areas and absent chest expansion with inhalations, provide additional clues. During apnea, when such spontaneous breathing movements are absent, complete airway obstruction can be recognized by the difficulty encountered to inflate the lungs when attempting to ventilate the patient. *Partial* airway obstruction is recognized by noisy air flow, which may also be accompanied by retraction. Snoring suggests that the partial obstruction is hypopharyngeal, due to the base of the tongue; crowing suggests laryngospasm; gurgling points to the presence of foreign matter; and wheezing signals bronchial obstruction.

The immediate sequelae of airway obstruction may also be suspected on clinical grounds. Hypercarbia, for example, is suspected when there is somnolence and is confirmed by measurement of increased arterial PCO_2. Hypoxemia is suspected when there is tachycardia, restlessness, sweating or cyanosis, and is confirmed by measurement of decreased arterial PO_2. Absence of cyanosis, however, does not rule out severe hypoxemia. Needless to say, during acute airway obstruction, attempts at clearing the airway and reoxygenation have absolute priority over arterial blood gas determinations.

Emergency Airway Control Measures (Table I)
Emergency oxygenation of the non-intubated patient is an art that is best acquired through guided clinical experience. Measures for emergency airway control are being improved continuously. Nonetheless, those described here have withstood the test of time. These measures should be practiced to perfection on manikins; it is then desirable to also practice on unconscious (anesthetized) patients under the direction of an experienced anesthesiologist.

When confronted with a seemingly unconscious patient in need of help, simultaneously with controlling the airway, do the following:
1 *Establish unreponsiveness* (gently shake and shout); and
2 *Call out for help.* Stay with the patient.

Recognition of acute airway obstruction must go hand in hand with therapeutic action, step by step, taking into account the number of personnel available, their training and the possible complications of various therapeutic maneuvers. The airway control measures (Table I) are intended primarily for the unconscious patient whose treatment requires rapid stepwise progression until the obstruction is controlled. Airway control measures 4, 5, 8 and 10 (Table I) may also be required for selected conscious patients.

Backward Tilt of Head (Fig. 2)
If the victim is unconscious, backward tilt of the head, forward displacement of the mandible, or both, prevent hypopharyngeal obstruction by the base of the tongue (Fig. 2—4). Either maneuver stretches the tissues between the larynx and mandible, and thereby lifts the base of the tongue from the posterior pharyngeal wall.

If he is unconscious place him/her in a supine position (face up) — and tilt his head backward by *neck lift,* i.e., with one hand under his neck and the other at his forehead (Fig. 2-B). This usually results in slight opening of his mouth.

If his mouth is closed or his chin is sagging (neck not stretched) — switch to *chin support,* by moving one hand from under his neck to hold the chin forward; hold his mouth slightly open, being careful not to compress the neck under the chin, as this causes obstruction (Fig. 2-C).

If dentures are firmly in place, leave them in position, for they maintain the contour of the mouth and make artificial ventilation somewhat easier; if they are loose, however, remove them.

Neck lift or chin support can be used interchangeably. Chin support does not displace the mandible forward. If airway obstruction persists, the mandible should be displaced forward (jaw thrust) and the mouth opened.

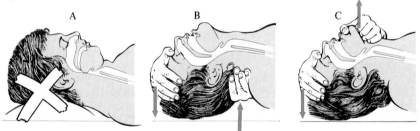

Figure 2: Backward tilt of head
(A) Hypopharyngeal obstruction by the tongue in coma with head in mid-position or flexed.
(B)(C) Backward tilt of the head stretches anterior neck structures and thereby lifts the base of the tongue off the posterior pharyngeal wall.
(B) Neck lift, which is easier to teach; and (C) chin support, which better controls opening of the mouth.

Positioning (Fig. 3)

The unconscious patient should be placed horizontally. Only when clearing the airway is required, transient head-down tilt may be used for gravity drainage of liquid foreign matter. However, avoid the prone (face-down) position, because it makes the face inaccessible, produces mechanical obstruction, and reduces thoracic compliance.

The *«supported supine aligned position»* (Fig. 3-A) is recommended for attended comatose patients in need of resuscitation. Elevation of the shoulders by a pillow or folded towel facilitates holding the head tilted backward. However, a pillow should never be placed under the head of the unconscious patient (as it flexes the neck forward, causing hypopharyngeal obstruction) except for tracheal intubation.

In cases of trauma, hold the head-neck-chest aligned (Fig. 3-A); provide only moderate, not maximal, backward tilt. Do not turn the victim's head laterally; do not flex his head forward. When the victim must be turned in order to clear his airway, hold his head-neck-chest aligned while another rescuer turns him.

The *«stable side position»* (Fig. 3-B) is recommended for the spontaneously breathing comatose patient, to promote gravity drainage of liquid foreign matter from the mouth. It is particularly important for mass casualties. This position is achieved by rolling the victim on his side, flexing his lower leg and placing his lower arm behind his back, with the hand of the upper arm under his chin to keep his head tilted backward. Support his head when you move him, so as not to aggravate a cervical spine injury. Some teach the stable side position as the first step after having determined unconsciousness, for airway clearing, to be followed by turning supine if artificial ventilation is needed.

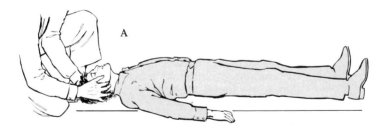

Figure 3: Positioning of the Unconscious Patient
(A) Supported supine aligned position — for resuscitation. Hold head, neck and chest aligned with slight traction. With both hands at sides of face, provide jaw thrust, open mouth and moderate backward tilt of head. Prevent flexion and rotation of head.

(B) Stable side position — for spontaneously breathing unconscious patient.

(1) Flex leg closest to you.

(2) Put hand closest to you under his buttocks.

(3) Gently roll him unto his side.

(4) Tilt his head backward and keep his face low. Put his upper hand under his lower cheek to maintain head-tilt and to prevent him from rolling onto his face. The lower arm behind his back prevents him from rolling backward.

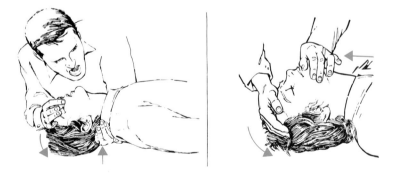

Figure 4: Techniques for backward tilt of head
Backward tilt of head, by neck-lift, plus positive pressure inflation with mouth-to-mouth (left) and mouth-to-nose (right) exhaled air inflations.

Positive Pressure Inflation Attempts (Fig. 4)
Emergency oxygenation attempts in the unconscious patient should start with backward tilt of the head (and in addition, if necessary, jaw thrust and opening of the mouth). If the airway remains obstructed — with or without breathing efforts — add positive pressure inflation attempts (Chapter 1B).

Assess airway patency and try to overcome obstruction by intermittent positive pressure inflation attempts — using exhaled air (e.g., mouth-to-mouth, mouth-to-nose, mouth-to-adjunct) (Fig. 4); air (e.g., self-refilling bag-valve-mask unit); or oxygen-enriched air (e.g., mouth- to-mask with oxygen, bag-valve-mask with oxygen). Adapt inflation patterns (pressure, volume, rate, rhythm and flow) according to patient efforts, airway-lung-chest resistances and gas leaks. If he is apneic, control ventilation by intermittent positive pressure (IPPV) or continuous positive pressure (CPPV). If there are spontaneous breathing movements, assist (augment) ventilation by intermittent positive pressure breathing (IPPB) or intermittent mandatory ventilation (IMV). For artificial ventilation techniques see Chapter 1B.

For the first few inflations in cardiac arrest, it has been suggested that positive end-expiratory pressure (PEEP) be added, by not letting the patient fully exhale («staircase» ventilation), in order to «recruit» collapsed or fluid-filled alveoli and thereby increase arterial PO_2. A sustained rise in intrathoracic pressure, however, can stop a feebly beating heart. Moreover, pressures which exceed $20-25$ cm H_2O can distend the stomach (Ruben) and thereby promote regurgitation. When higher pressures are needed, tracheal intubation is desirable. When the patient's muscles are not in spasm, a helper can prevent gastric regurgitation and insufflation by holding the cricoid cartilage of the larynx pressed backward to occlude the esophagus (Sellick).

Triple Airway Maneuver (Head Tilt, Mouth Open, Jaw Thrust) (Fig. 5)
In about 20% of unconscious patients, backward tilt of the head is not by itself sufficient to open the air passage. In such circumstances, additional forward displacement of the mandible is required to establish a patent airway (Esmarch, Heiberg, Safar). Even using these two maneuvers together there may occur expiratory nasopharyngeal obstruction in about one-third of unconscious patients, when the mouth is closed. For this reason the mouth should be held slightly open. In this regard, it is important to note that when the mouth is widely opened some stretch of the neck is lost, with consequent return of partial or complete hypopharyngeal obstruction. The necessary degree of stretch can, however, be regained by forward displacement of the mandible (jaw thrust) (Morikawa). Resulting pull on laryngeal muscles ameliorates

«laryngospasm» (Fink). The foregoing observations led to development of the «triple airway maneuver» — the combination of: (a) backward tilt of the head; (b) opening of the mouth; (c) forward displacement of the mandible (jaw thrust) — as the ideal manual method for producing supralaryngeal upper airway patency (Safar) (Fig. 5). Despite the fact that this maneuver is technically difficult, studies have shown that it can be taught to and mastered by lay personnel (Breivik, Esposito).

If the patient's breathing is spontaneous, position yourself at his vertex (Fig. 5-A). Grasp the ascending rami of his mandible in front of his ear lobes, using fingers 2—5 (or 2—4) of both hands and pull forcibly upwards (forwards), displacing the mandible so that the lower teeth jut out in front of the upper teeth («two-hands jaw lift»; «jaw thrust»). Retract the lower lip with your thumbs. Do not grasp the horizontal ramus of the mandible as this may close the mouth.

This procedure is painful and, for that reason, not only provides a patent airway but also serves as a useful test for the depth of unconsciousness; the patient who makes no purposeful response to the maneuver can safely be assumed to be in coma.

For direct mouth-to-mouth ventilation using head-tilt plus jaw thrust, position yourself at the side of the patient's head (Fig. 5-B). Readjust your hands to a comfortable position (e.g. your elbows resting on the ground), encircle his mouth widely with your lips, and occlude his nose with your cheek when blowing. For mouth-to-nose ventilation, encircle the entire nose with your lips and occlude his mouth with your other cheek or your thumb.
In the relaxed patient you can also perform jaw thrust effectively, displacing his mandible forward with your thumb in his mouth («thumb jaw lift») (Fig. 5-C). Do not use this method if he is responsive, as he may bite your thumb. During mouth-to-mouth breathing it may be difficult to obtain a good seal with your lips around your thumb.

In patients with suspected neck injury, in whom maximal backward tilt of the head might aggravate a spinal cord injury (flexion and rotation of the head are absolutely contraindicated), jaw thrust with moderate backward tilt of the head is the best method of airway control short of endotracheal intubation.

Backward tilt of the head, jaw thrust and opening of the mouth can be practiced on manikins, patients and co-workers.

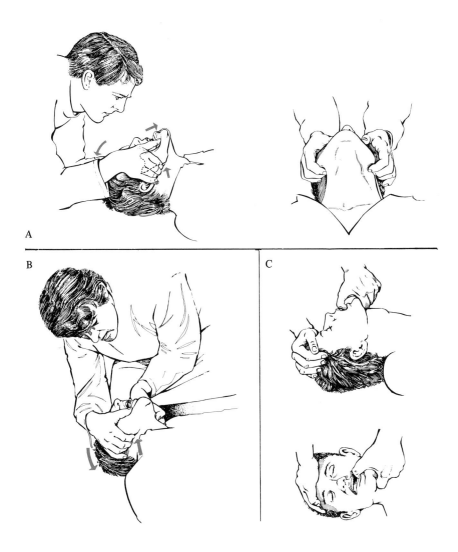

Figure 5: *Triple airway maneuver*
Tilt head backward, displace mandible forward and open mouth.

(A) With operator at patient's vertex, for spontaneously breathing patients. See text.

(B) With operator at side of patient for direct mouth-to-mouth ventilation. Seal nose with your cheek for mouth-to-mouth breathing. Seal mouth with your other cheek for mouth-to-nose breathing.

(C) Modified triple airway maneuver by thumb-jaw lift method (for relaxed patient only).

Manual Clearing of the Airway (Fig. 6)

When positive pressure inflation attempts meet obstruction in spite of backward tilt of the head, opening of the mouth and jaw thrust, and you suspect foreign matter in the upper airway, the mouth must be forced open and cleared of foreign material.

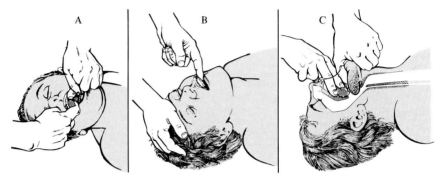

Figure 6: Three methods to force the mouth open for clearing, finger sweeping, suctioning, and inserting of airways or laryngoscope
(A) «Crossed-finger maneuver» for the moderately relaxed jaw.
(B) «Finger behind teeth maneuver» for the tight jaw.
(C) «Tongue-jaw-lift maneuver» for the very relaxed jaw.

1 *Force mouth open*, using one of the following three maneuvers:
A. The «crossed-finger maneuver» (Fig. 6-A) for the moderately relaxed jaw (Safar). Position yourself at the top or the side of the patient's head. Insert your index finger into the corner of his mouth, and press your index finger against his upper teeth; then press your thumb, crossed over your index finger, against his lower teeth, thereby forcing the mouth open. To leave ample room for instrumentation, be sure to insert your fingers into the far corner of the patient's mouth.
B. The «finger behind teeth maneuver» (Fig. 6-B) for the tight jaw (Safar). Insert one index finger between the patient's cheek and teeth and wedge the tip of you index finger behind his last molar teeth.
C. The «tongue-jaw-lift maneuver» (Fig. 6-C) for the fully relaxed jaw (Gordon). Insert your thumb into the patient's mouth and throat, and with the tip of your thumb lift the base of his tongue. The other fingers grasp the mandible at the chin and lift anteriorly.
    The above maneuvers for forcing the mouth open are also needed for suctioning, and insertion of airway and laryngoscope.

2 *Sweep one or two fingers* (perhaps covered with a piece of cloth) through mouth and pharynx for clearing (Fig. 6-A). Wipe out liquid

foreign matter with the index and middle fingers. Try to extract solid foreign matter from the pharynx with hooked index finger or using index plus middle fingers like tweezers (Fig. 6-C).

3 *Drain liquid foreign matter* by turning the head to the side. In accident victims turning the head to the side or flexing it forward must be avoided, since this may aggravate a spinal cord injury. If head turning is necessary in accident victims, the entire patient should be turned as a unit, with an assistant holding head, neck and chest in alignment (Fig. 3).

Blows and Thrusts for Foreign Body Obstruction (Fig. 7, 8, 9)
These are controversial techniques. The estimated death rate from inhaled or swallowed objects in the U.S.A. is 3000 cases per year, but the incidence seems less in other countries. Since few of these cases have had autopsy proof of foreign body obstruction, sudden cardiac death may be the cause of many of these deaths (Haugen).

In witnessed foreign body aspiration when the patient is conscious and *partially* obstructed, he should be encouraged to cough and spit it out, but digital probing, thrusts and blows should be avoided, as such maneuvers may aggravate the obstruction. The patient should be taken rapidly to the nearest hospital or physician, with oxygen inhalation en route.

In witnessed foreign body aspiration when the patient is conscious or unconscious, either with cyanosis, an ineffective cough, or *completely* obstructed (unable to cough), any possibly effective measure is justified as an act of desperation. No single method should be taught to the exclusion of others. Sudden complete obstruction can cause unconsciousness from hypoxemia within 1 — 2 minutes.

Severe foreign body obstruction is suspected: (1) in the conscious patient when he is suddenly unable to speak or cough and/or uses the distress signal for choking (e.g., clutching his neck) (Fig. 7-A); (2) in the unconscious patient when in spite of upper airway control the lungs cannot be inflated; and (3) when foreign body inhalation has been witnessed.

The optimal methods for relieving airway obstruction due to aspiration of a foreign body require *adjunctive equipment* — e.g., a laryngoscope, or tongue blade and flashlight, for visualization of the mouth, pharynx and larynx; forceps or suction for extraction of the foreign body under direct vision; and, if complete obstruction persists, equipment for cricothyrotomy or translaryngeal jet insufflation. However, such equipment should be deployed only by *health care professionals* trained in its use.

Blind extraction attempts with instruments are hazardous. There are no data to support the use of devices for foreign body extraction without visualization, such as the «Choke Saver» or «Throat-E-Vac».

For use by *lay personnel,* on the other hand, particularly in the conscious choking patient, *back blows* have been recommended for some time, but studied only recently (Gordon). *Abdominal thrusts* (Heimlich) have been promoted recently by the originator and were added to the CPR sequences. Recommendations for these thrust techniques are based on anecdotal evidence from conscious patients with sudden complete foreign body obstruction who ejected the foreign body when abdominal thrusts were used. However, there is also anecdotal evidence of failures with this technique (Redding).

Physiologic evidence indicates that back blows and abdominal and chest thrusts produce very weak increases in airway pressure when the airway is closed (blows are better than thrusts) and only slow air flow rates when the airway is open (thrusts are better than blows). Neither produce pressures or flows as effective as those created by natural cough (Gordon, Guildner, Ruben), and this difference may be accentuated in the choking patient who obstructs, after a cough spell, with a low residual lung volume.

Potential *complications* of abdominal thrusts include gastric rupture, injury to the liver and other organs, and induction of regurgitation. *Chest thrusts,* which are essentially the same as external cardiac compressions, may be safer. For this reason, some favor chest thrusts over abdominal thrusts for the unconscious patient (Guildner). Chest thrusts may induce ventricular fibrillation in the hypoxic sick heart. For the *techniques* of blows and thrusts, see legends to Fig. 7, 8, 9.

The following *sequence* is recommended Fig. 6, 7, 8, 9):

1 If the patient is *conscious,* encourage him to remove the foreign body himself by coughing. If this fails within seconds, ask him to open his mouth (if he is unconscious, force his mouth open) and sweep the mouth and pharynx with your hooked finger or with suction (Fig. 6).

Some agencies do not recommend finger probe for the conscious victim. Trained personnel with equipment should use a laryngoscope (or flashlight and tongue blade) and forceps (Magill forceps or Kelly clamp) for extraction of the foreign body under direct vision.

2 If the above method fails —
   (a) for the *conscious* patient, apply 3—5 back blows (Fig. 7-A) followed by 3—5 abdominal or chest thrusts (Fig. 7-B) and repeat clearing attempts (Fig. 6).
   (b) for the *unconscious* patient, place him horizontal and attempt to ventilate the lungs (slow forceful inflations can often force air around the foreign body). If this fails, apply 3—5 back blows (Fig. 8-A), followed by 3—5 abdominal thrusts (Fig. 8-B) or chest thrusts (identical with external cardiac compressions). Repeat clearing and ventilation attempts. If this also fails, repeat the sequence of

ventilation, back blows, chest thrusts, finger sweeps — until you succeed in ventilating the patient or until equipment for extraction under direct vision becomes available.

During ventilation attempts, jaw thrust may help alleviate the obstruction by widening the hypopharynx.

Check for the pulse; if pulseless, add CPR to clearing attempts.

3 As a final measure, cricothyrotomy or translaryngeal oxygen jet insufflation may be used if trained personnel and equipment are available.

Do *not* use abdominal thrusts in infants and in small children, because of the danger of injuring the liver, nor in pregnant women.

Documentation, however, of the superiority of the above over other possible combinations of methods is lacking. Some do not teach blows or thrusts.

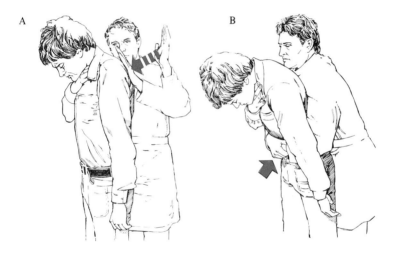

Figure 7: Back blows (A) and abdominal thrusts (B) for foreign body obstruction in the conscious standing or sitting victim

For back blows (A) deliver a series of 3—5 sharp blows with the heel of your hand over the victim's spine between the shoulder blades. If possible lower his head below his chest to utilize gravity.

For abdominal thrusts (B) stand behind the victim, wrap your arms around his waist, grasp your fist or wrist of one hand with the other, place your hands against his abdomen between navel and xiphoid process (rib cage), — and press your fist into his abdomen with a quick thrust upward. Repeat up to 3—5 times. Avoid the xyphoid process.

Less potentially injurious (particularly in pregnant or obese patients) are chest thrusts over the lower sternum (not shown).

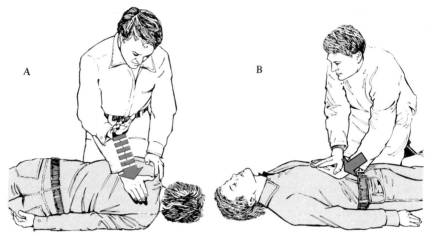

Figure 8: Back blows (A) and abdominal thrusts (B) for foreign body obstruction in the unconscious lying (horizontal) victim

For back blows (A) roll the victim on his side facing you, with his chest against your knees; deliver 3—5 sharp blows with the heel of your hand over the victim's spine, between the shoulder blades.

For abdominal thrusts (B) place the victim supine (face-up); kneel at the side of his abdomen or straddling it. Place one of your hands on top of the other, with the heel of the bottom hand in the midline between the patient's navel and xiphoid process. Lean forward so that your shoulders are over the victim's abdomen, and press toward the diaphragm with a quick thrust inward and upward. Do not press to the right or left of the midline. Repeat up to 3—5 times if necessary.

Less potentially injurious (particularly in pregnant or obese patients) are chest thrusts over the sternum (not shown), which are performed like external cardiac compressions.

Figure 9: Back blows in infants and small children

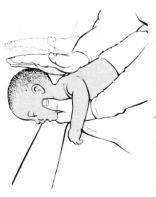

Hold the child facedown, supporting chin and neck with your knee and one hand, and apply gentle back blows between the shoulder blades. For chest thrusts (not shown), place the child face up on your forearm, lower his head, and apply chest thrusts gently with 2 or 3 fingers, as in external cardiac compressions. If the child's airway is only partially obstructed and he is conscious and able to breathe in the upright position, do not turn him head down. Do not use abdominal thrusts in infants and in small children.

Clearing the Airway by Suction (Fig. 10)

Suction has not been listed together with manual clearing because it requires equipment.

Suction devices include a vacuum source, a yoke with control valve, a nonbreakable collection bottle, a large-bore, non-kinking connecting tube, sterile suction tips and catheters of various sizes, water for rinsing and a suction trap (Fig. 10).

Equipment for *pharyngeal suction* should be powerful enough to clear semisolid foreign matter. Ideally it should produce a negative gauge pressure of at least 300 mm Hg when the tube is occluded, and air flow of at least 30 liters per minute when the tube is open (Rosen). Wall suction can be that forceful; portable suction units, on the other hand, are a compromise, as none meet the specifications.

Less suction force is required for *tracheobronchial suction* in adults and even less for pharyngeal and tracheobronchial suction in children and infants. For tracheobronchial suction, the force should be controllable, to avoid lung injury and asphyxia from lung collapse.

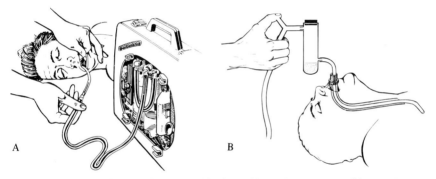

Figure 10: Suctioning by controllable wall suction or portable suction
(A) of oro-pharynx, with rigid tonsil suction tip; (B) of nasopharynx or tracheo-bronchial tree with curved-tip soft catheter.

For suction of *mouth and oropharynx*, use a tonsil suction device (Fig. 10-A). This is a rigid (metal or plastic) suction «tip» with multiple holes at the end. Force the mouth open with any of the maneuvers shown in Fig. 6, and sweep the suction tip through mouth and pharynx. Suction each nostril separately while occluding the other nostril.

For suction of the *tracheobronchial* tree and *nasopharynx* use a well-lubricated, soft, curved-tip catheter (Fig. 10-B). The curved tip permits deliberate insertion into one or the other main bronchus, whereas straight catheters usually pass only into the right main bronchus because of its lesser angle with the trachea. Insertion via tracheal or tracheostomy tube into the left main bronchus can also be enhanced by turning the head to the right. Choose a tracheobronchial suction catheter of a diameter which leaves room between suction catheter and wall of the tracheal tube through which it is inserted, so that air can enter the lungs during suctioning. Use tracheal suction tubes with a T or Y tube or lateral opening for on-off control. For tracheobronchial and nasal suctioning insert the catheter without suction and withdraw with rotation. Use a suction trap for inspection and examination of the suctioned material (Fig. 10B).

Blind nasotracheal suction attempts in the nonintubated patient call for the sitting sniffing position with raised occiput, head tilted backward and leaning forward. After topical anesthesia of the nasal passage, a well-lubricated, curved-tip catheter is inserted during a deep inhalation, while the tongue is pulled forward with a piece of dry gauze. This technique is safe only in the conscious, cooperative patient. However, in stupor or coma it may produce intractable laryngospasm, vomiting with aspiration, and asphyxial or reflex cardiac arrest.

Pharyngeal Intubation (Fig. 11)
Nasopharyngeal and oropharyngeal tubes, commonly known as «airways», hold the base of the tongue forward and counter obstruction by lips, teeth, and nose. Thus they can be substituted for two components of the triple airway maneuver — jaw thrust and opening of the mouth — which are not easily maintained over long periods. Even with the pharyngeal tube in place, however, the third component of the triple airway maneuver — backward tilt of the head — is still required. This is because, with flexion of the neck, the tip of the tube becomes partially withdrawn and the base of the tongue is pressed against the posterior pharyngeal wall and between the tip of the tube and the laryngeal entrance. An occasional patient may also require jaw thrust in spite of the pharyngeal tube.

Airways should be inserted into comatose patients only, as these devices may provoke laryngospasm or vomiting in persons with intact upper airway reflexes. Shortened airways, however, can be improvised to serve as mouth props (bite blocks) in conscious or stuporous patients. Nasopharyngeal tubes can cause epistaxis, which however can be minimized by use of a soft tube and correct technique. Advantages of the nasopharyngeal over the oropharyngeal tube include ability to insert the tube also in patients with trismus or clenched jaws and better tolerance even in the marginally stuporous patient. The oropharyngeal tube provides a wider airway.

Nasopharyngeal tubes should be of very soft rubber or plastic (Fig. 11-A). Insert the well-lubricated (preferably with anesthetic water- soluble lubricant) tube parallel to the level of the palate, until you feel the «give» of the angle of the nasopharyngeal air passage. Then advance the tube until air flow is optimal. Too deep insertion may cause laryngospasm or entry into the upper esophagus. Check air flow before securing the tube with tape.

Oropharyngeal tubes are of the Guedel type (Fig. 11-B). They come in several sizes (large adult, adult, child, infant, newborn) and are made of rubber, plastic, or metal. For resuscitation, at least 3 sizes (adult, child, infant) should be on hand. For insertion, first force the mouth open with the crossed-finger, tongue-jaw-lift or finger-behind-teeth maneuver (Fig. 6). Then insert the tube *over* the tongue (Fig. 11-B). This can be accomplished either by first inserting the tube into the mouth with curve reversed (convexity caudad) and then rotating it into its proper position, or by using a tongue blade to depress the tongue while the tube is slid past it. Incorrect placement of an oropharyngeal tube can push the tongue back into the pharynx and produce airway obstruction. Forceful insertion of a pharyngeal tube must also be avoided. Teeth can easily be damaged. Lips should not be caught between teeth and tube.

S-tubes are S-shaped mouth-to-mouth airways, which can be reversed to provide 2 sizes each (Fig. 11-C) (Safar). The operator prevents leakage of air with one hand pinching the nose and the other sealing the flange against the lips; or with the thenar eminences of both thumbs pinching the nose, the tips of both thumbs sealing the flange, and the fingers pulling on the ascending rami of the mandible.

A

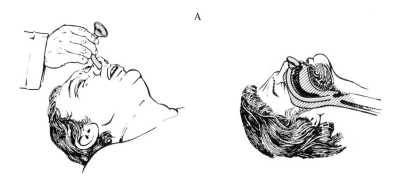

Figure 11: Nasopharyngeal and oropharyngeal tubes (airways)
(A) Nasopharyngeal tube. Insert well-lubricated tube into patent nasal passage (parallel to palate) until tip rests in hypopharynx (indicated by good air flow).

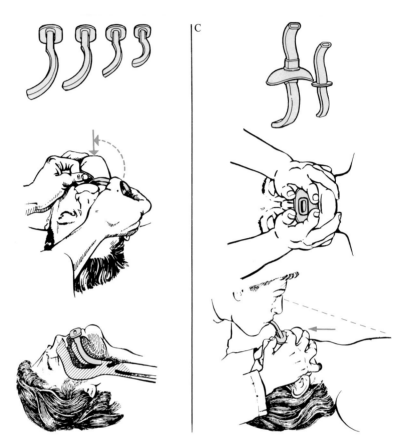

Figure 11, (continued)

*(B) Regular oropharyngeal tubes. Insert only if the jaw is moderately relaxed. Force the mouth open and insert tube **over** the tongue with 180-degree rotation, without pushing the base of the tongue backward. Alternatively, use tongue blade without turning airway. The tip should lie in the hypopharynx.*

(C) S-shaped mouth-to-mouth oropharyngeal tubes (adult-child size; child-infant size). Insert like regular oropharyngeal tube. Seal flange and nose. Tilt head backward. Inflate lungs as described in Chapter 1B.

Esophageal Obturator Airway Insertion (Fig. 12)

The esophageal obturator airway (Don Michael) is used to prevent gastric regurgitation and gastric insufflation during positive pressure artificial ventilation. The name of the device is somewhat misleading, for the device does not itself maintain a patent airway, but merely obstructs the esophagus, thereby preventing reflux of gastric contents into the pharynx.

It does not, however, obviate the need to maintain backward tilt of the head, nor does it in any way provide definitive control over or protection of the airway. Thus it should not be considered a substitute for endotracheal intubation, but rather should be viewed as an alternative to a simple mask device. Because its insertion is relatively easy and does not require visualization of the larynx, it can be used by personnel not trained in or not permitted to perform endotracheal intubation, and indeed it has been used by paramedics in large series of cardiac arrest cases outside hospitals (Gordon, Schofferman).

The esophageal obturator airway is a large-bore tube, approximately the size of a tracheal tube, with a rounded closed tip distally, a cuff to be inflated in the esophagus, and multiple openings at the hypopharyngeal level through which air or oxygen is delivered by intermittent positive pressure into the larynx and trachea. A modification, the esophageal gastric tube airway (Gordon) uses the lumen of the tube for gastric drainage; it therefore is without openings at the pharyngeal level and provides ventilation through an additional port in the mask, utilizing the nasal passage (which may be obstructed).

Insert an esophageal obturator airway only in deeply comatose patients! Its use is contraindicated in children under 16, in patients who have swallowed caustic agents or in patients with any known history of esophageal disease.

Attach the mask to the proximal end of the tube. Open the patient's mouth and hold his mandible and tongue forward with your thumb (Fig. 12-A). Insert the esophageal obturator airway through the patient's mouth into the esophagus while the patient's head is held in slight flexion. Confirm correct positioning of the tube and inflate the esophageal cuff. Seal the mask against the patient's face and ventilate by mouth or bag-valve unit (Fig. 12-B). During ventilation hold his head tilted backward.

When a patient is delivered to the Emergency Department with an esophageal obturator airway in place and is deeply comatose, the trachea should be intubated with a cuffed tube prior to removal of the esophageal obturator airway. Be prepared to suction regurgitated material which appears immediately upon removal of the esophageal obturator airway.

If the patient is recovering reflexes, leave the esophageal obturator airway in place until he is conscious and breathing spontaneously or at least has recovered protective upper airway reflexes, since removal may be followed by massive regurgitation. Physicians and nurses working in Emergency Departments must be familiar with this device and the proper timing and technique of its removal.

Complications of esophageal obturator airway insertion have occurred primarily in spontaneously breathing patients who were not deeply comatose. Injuries encountered include esophageal rupture, asphyxia from inadvertent tracheal intubation (which seems to occur in almost 10% of the cases, but is of no consequence if immediately recognized), and provocation of laryngospasm, vomiting, and aspiration. Use of the device should be restricted to adequately trained personnel. The main drawbacks to its use are inability to control laryngospasm, suction the tracheobronchial tree or protect the lungs against aspiration of foreign matter or blood from the upper airway.

Esophageal obturator airway insertion is a poor substitute for, not an alternative to, tracheal intubation. For paramedics, endotracheal intubation should be a mandatory skill, and esophageal obturator airway insertion only an optional skill (Caroline).

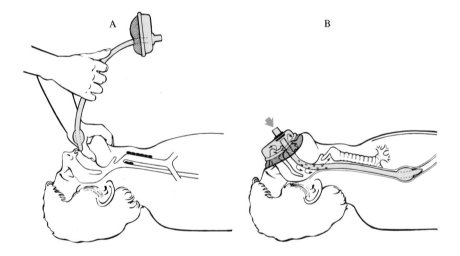

Figure 12: Esophageal obturator airway

For insertion only into relaxed, apneic adult patient, by personnel unable to perform tracheal intubation.

(A) Blind insertion via mouth into esophagus. For insertion keep neck slightly flexed.

(B) Correct position for intermittent positive pressure ventilation. For ventilation keep head tilted backward. See text.

Tracheal Intubation (Fig. 13, 14, 15; Table II)

An endotracheal tube can isolate the airway, keep it patent, prevent aspiration, and facilitate ventilation, oxygenation and suctioning. The technique of endotracheal intubation, which has revolutionized anesthesia and resuscitation, was pioneered by many, including Chaillou, Kuhn, Magill, Macintosh, Gillespie, Waters and Deming.

Endotracheal intubation is *indicated* as the final option of emergency airway control in *unconscious* patients. It is indicated in most comatose patients unless they are so light that upper airway reflexes are intact, coma is expected to be brief in duration, and the patient is attended continuously by personnel experienced with airway control in the unintubated patient. As a guide, the patient who tolerates an intubation attempt needs a tracheal tube.

Endotracheal intubation is also indicated in the *conscious* patient with: (1) inadequate spontaneous clearing of the tracheobronchial tree; (2) suspected aspiration; (3) absence of laryngeal reflexes; or (4) need for prolonged mechanical ventilation. After 7 to 10 days a switch to tracheotomy should be considered, earlier in selected cases. Improved cuffs (Carroll) and tubes (Lindholm) have minimized laryngotracheal damage. Thus, in comatose patients, tracheotomy may be delayed if extubation is expected to be possible in $1-2$ weeks. Selected conscious patients in need of prolonged intratracheal ventilation, however, may be more comfortable and be given the opportunity to talk, if switch to a tracheotomy is performed earlier.

Manual airway control, ventilation and oxygenation attempts without equipment or simple adjuncts should always precede attempts at tracheal intubation. During CPR, however, lung inflations accompanying heart compressions require high pharyngeal pressures which may cause gastric insufflation. This can promote regurgitation and aspiration. Therefore, during CPR, the trachea should be intubated as soon as possible, but only after adequate preoxygenation and without interrupting cardiac compressions for more than 15 seconds at a time. Once the tracheal tube has been inserted, lung inflations do not have to be synchronized with chest compressions.

Tracheal intubation may be performed through the mouth or through the nose. Orotracheal intubation is preferable in an emergency situation, since it can be accomplished more rapidly and with less trauma than nasotracheal intubation.

Equipment for Tracheal Intubation (Fig. 13, Table II)

The equipment needed for laryngoscopy, extraction of foreign bodies and tracheal intubation should be in every prehospital life support station, ambulance, emergency department, ICU, and other selected hospital locations. Details depend on individual preference. Immediate readiness is important. All equipment should be checked frequently, for patency of tracheal tube, cuffs, adequacy of laryngoscope batteries, etc.

TABLE II A
Approximate sizes of endo-tracheal and tracheostomy tubes

Approximate age	Weight (kg)	+ Outside diameter (mm)	French size (Circumference)	Magill sizes	Length of tube (cm)** OT	NT	Suction catheters (French sizes)	+ Adapters mm ID	Shiley	Aberdeen	Holinger	Approx length (mm)
		14.0	42									
		13.3	40		22-26	29	14					
Adult male		13.0	39									
		12.7	38	10	22-26	29	14					60
(French 34-40)		12.3	37									
		12.0	36		22-26	29	14					
Adult female		11.7	35	9								
		11.3	34		20-24	27	12					60
(French 32-36)		11.0	33									
		10.7	32	8	20-24	27	12					
12-13 yrs.		10.7	32	8	19	25	10	9	6	7.0	6	60
		10.3	31	7	19	25	10	9	6	7.0	6	
10-11 yrs.		10.0	30		18	24	10	9	6	6.0	6	60
		9.7	29	6	18	24	10	9	6	6.0	6	
8-9 yrs.		9.3	28	5½	17	22½	10	8	4	6.0	5	55
		9.0	27	5	17	22½	10	8	4	6.0	5	
6-7 yrs.		8.7	26	4½	15	22	10	7	4	5.0	4	55
		8.3	25	4	15	22	10	7	4	5.0	4	
4-5 yrs.	16–20	8.0	24	3½	14	18½	10	7	4	5.0	4	50
		7.7	23	3	14	18½	8	7	4	5.0	4	
2-3 yrs.	11–15	7.3	22	2½	13	17	8	6	4	5.0	4	50
		7.0	21	2	13	17	8	6	4	5.0	4	
1-2 yrs.	9–11	6.7	20	1½	12	15½	8	6	3	5.0	3	45
		6.3	19	1	12	15½	8	6	3	5.0	3	
3-12 mos.	5–9	6.0	18		11	14	8	5	2	4.5	3	45
		5.7	17		10	12½	6	5	1	4.0	2	
Newborn - 3 mos.	2.5–5	5.3	16	0	10	12	6	5	0	3.5	1	40
		5.0	15		10	11½	6	4	0	3.5	1	
Newborn	2–2.5	4.7	14		9½	10½	6	4	0	3.5	0	30
		4.3	13	00	8	9	6	3	0	3.5	0	
Premature	1–2	4.0	12		8	9	6	3	00		00	<30
		3.7	11		8	9	6	2	00		00	

* For adults and large children, tubes with large-volume soft cuffs are recommended; for children under 6 years of age, uncuffed tubes. For nasotracheal tubes select 1 mm outside diameter (2-3 French size) smaller than for orotracheal intubation.

** The lengths of pediatric orotracheal tubes given here are purposely short, to be used with the adapter within the mouth. OT = orotracheal: NT = nasotracheal.

+ Inside diameter (ID) is 1-4 mm less than outside diameter (OD), depending on wall thickness of tube.

Anesthesiologists, critical care physicians, emergency physicians and ambulance personnel should be able to intubate the trachea with both the straight (Magill) and the curved (Macintosh) blade (Fig. 13). The straight blade is designed to pick up the epiglottis directly, while the curved blade, which slips into the vallecula just above the epiglottis, lifts the epiglottis off the larynx indirectly, by pulling on the glosso-epiglottic frenulum. The curved blade does not touch the larynx itself and therefore probably produces less trauma and less reflex stimulation; it also permits more room for viewing and for tube insertion. Intubation in children requires special pediatric laryngoscope blades (Table II B).

Most endotracheal tubes as supplied are too long and must be cut (Table II A). The length of tube needed can be estimated by placing it alongside the patient's face and neck, with the bifurcation of the trachea being at the manubrio-sternal junction. The appropriate tube diameters are critical, particularly in selecting tubes for children (Table II A), but can be estimated from the diameter of the child's little finger. For resuscitation trays an assortment of 6 — 10 tube diameters (between 12 and 38 French sizes) is adequate.

For adults and children over 6 years, tubes with large-volume, low-pressure soft cuffs are recommended; for infants and small children, uncuffed tubes are better. Narrow small-volume, high-pressure cuffs should not be used because they may cause necrosis of the tracheal mucosa (Hedden). Overinflation of the cuff can be avoided by monitoring intracuff pressure (which in large soft cuffs equals airway and tracheal wall pressure) (Carroll) or by use of a pressure-limiting balloon. The tubes should be made of nonirritating plastic. Those reinforced with coiled wire are less likely to kink or be compressed, but are more difficult to insert. All tubes must have standard 15 mm male fittings.

TABLE II B

Laryngoscope Blades

Size	Straight Blade		Curved Blade	
	Length (mm)	Example	Length (mm)	Example
Adult (large)	190	Flagg No. 4	158	Macintosh No. 4
Adult (medium)	160	Flagg No. 3	130	Macintosh No. 3
Child (2–9 yrs.)	133	Flagg No. 2	108	Macintosh No. 2
Child (3 mo.–2 yrs.)	115	Wis-Hipple No. 1-1/2	100	Macintosh No. 1
Infant (under 3 mo.)	102	Flagg No. 1, Miller Infant		
Premature	75	Miller Premature		

TABLE II C

Rigid Tube Bronchoscopes
(use ventilation attachment)

Age	Inside Diameter (mm)	Length (cm)
Adult (large)	9	40
Adult (medium)	7	40
Child (5–8 yrs.)	5	30–33
Child (1–4 yrs.)	4	26
Infant (under 1 yr.)	3	26

A blunt-tipped metal or plastic malleable stylet makes the curvature of the tube controllable. When used it should not protrude beyond the distal end of the tube. Use of a straight stylet, bent 45° at the distal fifth of its length (hockey stick configuration), together with a curved laryngoscope blade facilitates intubation under difficult circumstances, even when only the rim of the epiglottis can be visualized.

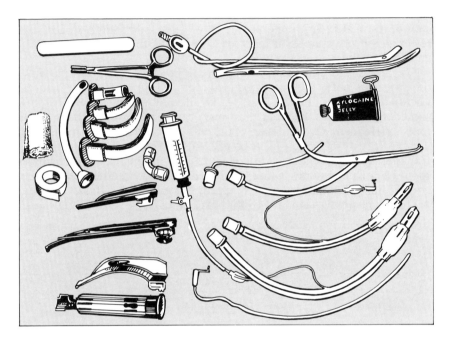

Figure 13: Equipment for tracheal intubation

On left, from top to bottom, tongue blade, clamp for cuff, bite block, tape to secure tracheal tube, nasopharyngeal tube, oropharyngeal tubes, curved connector, laryngoscope handle with adult curved and straight blades and child straight blade. At right, from top to bottom, curved-tip tracheal suction catheter, pharyngeal rigid suction tip, lidocaine water-soluble jelly. Magill forceps, three-way stopcock and syringe for cuff inflation, assortment of tracheal tubes (sizes French 12 infant — 38 adult), stylet. (See text).

Technique of Orotracheal Intubation (Fig. 14,15)

Intubation techniques are best learned by observing and practicing in the nonemergency setting. Equally important as insertion of the tube into the trachea are the many ancillary steps before and after intubation. Technique is influenced by personal preference, but should in any event be orderly, systematic and well-rehearsed.

The following sequence of action is recommended, which should be learned by supervised practice to perfection, first on adult and infant intubation manikins and then on anesthetized patients:

1 Have an assistant available if possible.

2 Select, prepare and check the equipment (Fig. 13). Do not depend on others.
   a Select the appropriate size tracheal tube (Table II A) and a spare tube one size smaller.
   b Select the appropriate size and type of laryngoscope (Table II B). Check the laryngoscope light.
   c Lubricate tracheal tube with a water-soluble anesthetic jelly, e.g., lidocaine (lignocaine, Xylocaine).
   d Check the cuff by manipulation of cuff pilot tube-stopcock-syringe assembly, and deflate the cuff.

3 Have the patient in the supine position, with the occiput elevated and the head tilted backward (sniffing position) to bring the laryngoscope blade and trachea into a straight line (Fig. 15).

4 Oxygenate the patient, preferably with 100 per cent O_2 for at least 2 minutes (e.g., with bag-valve-mask-oxygen) if feasible.

5 Interrupt ventilation for intubation. When intubating an apneic patient, hold your own breath and stop the intubation attempt when you become short of breath.

6 For insertion of the tube —
   a First force the patient's mouth open with your right hand (e.g., with crossed-finger maneuver) (Fig. 6).
   b Grasp the laryngoscope handle firmly with the left hand, and insert the blade from the right corner of the patient's mouth, pushing his tongue to the left, so as not to obscure the view by the tongue bulging over the open side of the laryngoscope blade (Fig. 15). Protect the lips from being injured between teeth and blade.
   c Move the laryngoscope blade toward the midline and visualize the patient's mouth, uvula, pharynx, and epiglottis (Fig. 14B) while moving your right hand to the patient's forehead or occiput to hold his head tilted backward.
   d Visualize the arytenoids and the midline (the most important

landmarks) (Fig. 14C), and finally the vocal cords (desirable but not essential) (Fig. 14D), by lifting the epiglottis directly with the straight blade (Fig. 15A) or indirectly with the curved blade (Fig. 15B).

e Expose the larynx by pulling the laryngoscope handle upward (forward) at a right angle to the blade. Do not use the upper teeth as a fulcrum. When using the curved blade, insertion too deep will push the epiglottis downward, whereas a too superficial insertion will make the base of the tongue bulge and obscure the vision of the larynx. Using the straight blade, insertion too deeply into the esophagus will lift the entire larynx out of view. These mistakes can be avoided by recognition of the arytenoid cartilages (Fig. 14C).

f If necessary, ask an assistant to push the larynx backwards for a better view (Fig. 14D). Ask him to retract the right corner of the mouth to gain space for tube insertion.

g Insert the tracheal tube (with your right hand) through the right corner of the patient's mouth, while looking through the laryngoscope blade (Fig. 15C). Twist the tube if necessary. Observe the tip of the tube and the cuff as they pass through the larynx and advance the tube so the cuff is placed just below the larynx.

h Ask the assistant to hold the tube in place against the corner of the patient's mouth.

7 Remove the stylet, if used, and immediately ventilate and oxygenate by a self-refilling bag-valve-oxygen unit or anesthesia circuit, and switch to a mechanical ventilator if desired, but only after the ability to ventilate has been ascertained by manual lung inflations.

8 Inflate the cuff (e.g., via three-way stopcock) temporarily, to achieve a seal to protect against aspiration.

9 Turn ventilation and oxygenation over to your assistant.

10 Remove the laryngoscope blade and insert an oropharyngeal tube or bite block.

11 Position the tube to avoid bronchial intubation, using one of the following steps:
   a Press with one finger into the suprasternal notch and feel for the tip of the tube; advance the tube with the other hand 2 cm further. Retain correct depth of tube insertion by marking tube length at level of upper teeth.
   b Auscultate both lungs to rule out bronchial (usually right bronchial) intubation; and to determine need for suctioning.

12 Tape the tube securely to the patient's face. When the cheeks are unshaven or moist, a dry, broad, loose tape can be placed around

neck and both cheeks first and the tube taped to it; or an umbilical tape placed loosely around the neck can be tied to the tube.

13 While applying continuous positive pressure, reinflate the cuff permanently, but only to the point of abolishing audible leaks. (Inflate large low pressure cuffs to 15 — 20 cm H_2O intracuff pressure between lung inflations).

14 Suction the tracheobronchial tree if necessary. If aspiration is suspected, use a suction trap for inspection and examination of the material removed (Fig. 10B).

15 Establish nonkinking, nonslipping connections to the ventilation-oxygenation device.

16 In a patient with deep coma or gastric distention, insert a gastric tube, preferably through the nose — if this proves impossible, through the mouth (see later).

17 During anesthesia, insert an esophageal stethoscope for monitoring of heart and breath sounds.

18 Deliver oxygen via a heated humidifier or nebulizer and use atraumatic aseptic suctioning as needed.

Rapid Intubation

The patient with a *full stomach* who is in need of general anesthesia or who is in coma from illness or injury may require *rapid («crash»)* *intubation* (Stept). Be prepared with suction for regurgitation. The choice between the supine and the semi-sitting position is controversial. The supine position (particularly if the head is lowered) may counteract aspiration, while the semi-sitting position may discourage possible regurgitation. After preoxygenation (preferably with 100% oxygen without positive pressure), close the patient's esophagus by pressure on the cricoid (Sellick) and paralyze the patient with succinylcholine. Intubate swiftly.

The convulsing, asphyxiated patient with head injury is a challenging example. He may have to be intubated with a muscle relaxant, since coughing and straining in the presence of brain contusion can cause additional cerebral edema and hemorrhage.

Crash intubation may be hazardous in the hands of the inexperienced.

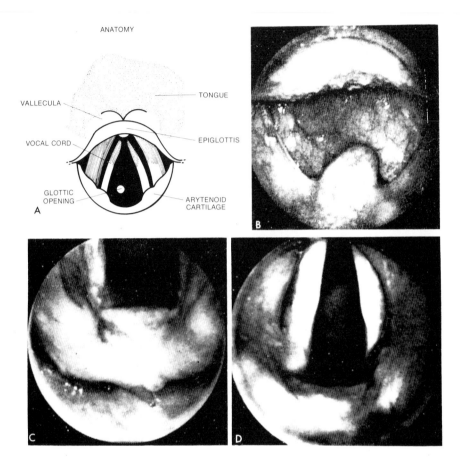

Figure 14: Anatomical views for endotracheal intubation

(A) Diagram of the anatomy of the laryngeal entrance exposed by direct laryngoscopy. (From American Heart Association Advanced Life Support Slide Series, 1976).

(B) First direct laryngoscopic view during tracheal intubation; exposure of uvula and epiglottis.

(C) Second direct laryngoscopic view during tracheal intubation; exposure of arytenoids.

(D) Third direct laryngoscopic view during tracheal intubation; exposure of glottis. The anterior commissure is not fully seen. The posterior commissure is below.

(Views B, C and D are from Holinger, P.H., et al.: J. Thorac. Surg. 17:178, 1948).

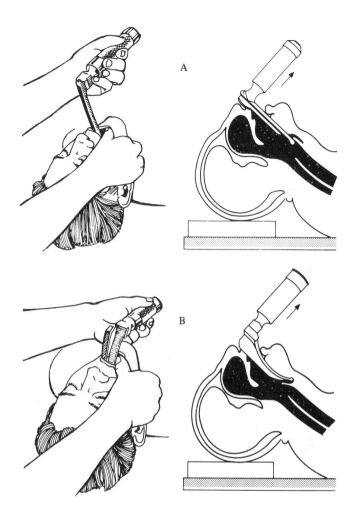

Figure 15: Technique of orotracheal intubation

(A) Laryngoscopy for endotracheal intubation with straight laryngoscope blade. **Left,** *insertion of blade;* **right,** *larynx exposed. Note elevated occiput with head tilted backward (sniffing position). Note direct elevation of epiglottis with tip of blade. (Do not use teeth as fulcrum.)*

(B) Laryngoscopy for endotracheal intubation with curved laryngoscope blade. **Left,** *insertion of blade;* **right,** *larynx exposed. Note indirect elevation of epiglottis by tip of blade elevating base of tongue.*

C

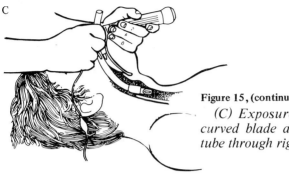

Figure 15, (continued)
(C) Exposure of the larynx with curved blade and insertion of cuffed tube through right corner of mouth.

Intubating the awake patient

Endotracheal intubation of the awake patient is thought by some to be *indicated* prior to general anesthesia in aspiration risks or severe pulmonary insufficiency; for upper airway and laryngoscopic procedures; and in selected cases for prolonged mechanical ventilation, as in patients with severe chest injury.

Tracheal intubation of the conscious patient is difficult and requires skill, experience, and artistry. Topical anesthesia of the upper airway mucosa is provided by spraying a topical anesthetic, e.g., 4 per cent lidocaine (lignocaine, Xylocaine) from a nebulizer, first onto the tongue and oropharyngeal mucosa, then under direct vision, with a partially inserted laryngoscope blade, onto the hypopharynx and supraglottic laryngeal mucosa, avoiding stimulation of the gag reflex.

The tracheal mucosa is then sprayed with 2-3 ml of 4 per cent lidocaine (lignocaine, Xylocaine) either by instillation through the glottis into the tracheal lumen using a cannula with multiple holes, or by translaryngeal injection through the cricothyroid membrane, using a thin (e.g., 22 gauge) needle.

The procedure may be facilitated by a sedative or analgesic by IV titration (e.g., diazepam, meperidine (pethidine, Demerol)). Take care not to abolish the response to verbal command. Suction should be ready to cope with regurgitation. For intubation the laryngoscope blade and tracheal tube must be handled securely, gently applying pressure only when and where absolutely necessary. The operator's reassuring voice is most important.

Should he regurgitate or vomit before the tube is inserted, suction and coach him to help clearing by coughing.

Technique of Nasotracheal Intubation

Nasotracheal intubation is more difficult, more time-consuming and potentially more traumatic (epistaxis) than orotracheal intubation. The blind nasotracheal technique is less predictable. Furthermore the technique carries the risk of introducing nasal bacteria into the trachea. It is not a suitable procedure for emergency airway control in the asphyxiating patient. However, in several circumstances in which the patient is breathing spontaneously and is not asphyxiated, e.g., in cases of tight jaw (trismus), or inability to tilt the head backward (suspected neck fracture), nasotracheal intubation may be required. It is also thought by many to be more suitable for long-term intubation, as the nasal tube is better tolerated than the oral tube.

For intubating through the patient's nose, select the patient's more patent nasal passage by checking his ability to sniff through each nostril separately. For intubating the *conscious* patient, apply a nasal vasoconstrictor (e.g. phenylephrine drops or spray) to dilate the nasal air passage, together with a topical anesthetic, e.g., 4 per cent lidocaine (lignocaine, Xylocaine) to minimize discomfort. Alternately, cocaine 1—2 per cent may be used in small amounts, as it is both a potent topical vasoconstrictor and anesthetic. Apply topical anesthesia to hypopharynx, larynx, and trachea as described above. Nasotracheal tubes should be very soft, well curved and well lubricated, cuffed for adults. The size should be 1 mm outside diameter (2-3 French sizes) smaller than for orotracheal intubation (Table II A).

Insert the tube through the more patent nostril, parallel to the palate. Ideally the tube's bevel should face the nasal septum to avoid damaging the turbinates. Tilt the patient's head backwards moderately and elevate the occiput. Advance the tube beyond the «give» of the nasopharyngeal angle.

For *blind* nasotracheal intubation, maneuver the tip of the tube laterally by twisting it, and maneuver it anteriorly or posteriorly by extending or flexing the head (not in suspected neck injury!). Then advance the tube during inhalations, listening for air flow or coughing that indicate entry into the larynx. If the patient's mouth can be opened, nasotracheal intubation can be facilitated by *visualizing* the larynx. In this case hold the laryngoscope in your left hand. Direct the tube, using Magill's forceps or a large Kelly clamp in your right hand to grasp the tube and guide it in the right direction, under direct vision — while your assistant advances the tube through the nose. This technique is also recommended for nasotracheal intubation in the *comatose* patient whose mouth can be opened.

Difficult Intubation
Intubation attempts may fail when there is inadequate muscular relaxation, poor technique, or anatomic abnormality. Difficulty with intubation can be anticipated, for example, when the patient has taut neck

tissues, a short thick neck, receding jaw, protruding teeth, inability to tilt the head backward, a narrow oral cavity, or a large tongue. In such patients, intubation should be attempted by the most skilled anesthesiologist immediately available.

Elective intubation in the spontaneously breathing, oxygenated patient, when difficulties with intubation are anticipated, can be accomplished with the use of a flexible fiberoptic laryngoscope or bronchoscope. The endotracheal tube to be used is inserted through the nose (preferable route) or mouth into the hypopharynx. The well-lubricated, flexible fiberoptic laryngoscope (with a diameter considerably smaller than that of the tracheal tube so that the patient can breathe around the scope) is inserted through the tube and directed under vision through the larynx into the trachea. When the tip of the flexible fiberoptic laryngoscope or bronchoscope enters the trachea, the tracheal tube is slipped over the flexible scope into the trachea, and the flexible scope is removed. For highly specialized intubation techniques or unusual circumstances, consult the anesthesia literature.

Tracheal Intubation in Infants and Small Children

When intubating the trachea in infants and small children, the operator must keep in mind that the infant's larynx in relation to that of the adult is located higher, has a floppy U-shaped epiglottis, and is funnel-shaped, with the narrowest diameter at the level of the cricoid ring. Selecting a tube with too large a diameter can cause croup with asphyxia from reactive narrowing at the cricoid level following extubation.

For intubation in infants, particularly in newborns, use of a straight pointed blade (e.g., Miller blade) is more satisfactory than the curved laryngoscope blade (Table II B). Since the small dimensions of the infant make accidental bronchial intubation more likely, we recommend for newborn resuscitation a tapered «Cole» tube, which has a shoulder at the larynx entrance, thus minimizing accidental bronchial intubation. For long-term use in infants, regular plastic tubes without shoulders are less injurious. Selecting the tube with the optimal diameter and length (Table II A), use of perfect atraumatic techniques, and attention to details are important.

Extubation

The technique of extubation is potentially hazardous, and its safe execution depends on special knowledge and skills. At the end of general anesthesia in the healthy person the endotracheal tube is removed either under sufficient depth of anesthesia to obviate postextubation laryngospasm or when the patient has recovered upper airway reflexes and responds to command. Respiratory insufficiency (hypoxemia, hypercarbia), acute acid-base abnormalities and circulatory derangements should be ruled out prior to extubation. Ideally, the patient should be conscious and able to achieve upon command an inspiratory capacity («sighing volume») of at least 15 ml/kg, to avoid progressive atelectasis after extubation. Other signs of recovered muscular power include ability to squeeze your hand, and to raise his head, and the absence of retractions during spontaneous breathing. Also, the stomach should not be distended.

The recommended *technique of extubation* requires an assistant. First, suction the patient's mouth, oropharynx and nasopharynx. Then allow the patient to breathe 100 % oxygen for 2—3 minutes and suction the tracheobronchial tree with a separate, sterile, curved-tip catheter. After suctioning, again allow the patient to breathe 100 per cent oxygen if time permits. Then, while you apply positive pressure to the trachea via bag-valve device, instruct your assistant to deflate the cuff of the endotracheal tube; the positive pressure helps to exsufflate secretions (which have accumulated above and below the cuff) into the pharynx, which should be suctioned promptly.

Having deflated the cuff, remove the tube gently while maintaining positive pressure with 100 per cent O_2 in the trachea. Tracheal suction should not be continued during withdrawal of the tracheal tube, as this can empty the lungs and cause severe hypoxemia. After removal of the tube, oxygenation is continued by mask, using approximately 50 % oxygen.

Be prepared to treat postextubation laryngospasm with oxygen by positive pressure and, if necessary, with a relaxant (i.e. succinylcholine) and reintubation. For extubation of patients with upper airway problems, cricothyrotomy equipment should be ready.

Complications of Tracheal Intubation

Attempts at endotracheal intubation can injure the lips, tongue, teeth, pharynx, tonsils and larynx. Nasotracheal intubation can cause epistaxis and, in addition, injure the nasal mucosa and the adenoids. Undetected, inadvertent intubation of the esophagus is the most dangerous complication of oro- and nasotracheal intubation attempts. Esophageal intubation may go unnoticed, unless one listens carefully for breath sounds over both sides of the chest and over the epigastrium. Other potential complications include: tube obstruction by compression, kinking, obstructing secretions, biting, a bulging cuff, a too-narrow lumen, or obstructing adapters; accidental bronchial intubation; and tube dislodgement. Persistent coughing (bucking, chest wall spasm) calls for positive pressure inflation with oxygen, and may require sedation, anesthesia, or even curarization to facilitate oxygenation and prevent asphyxia.

Long-term complications following extubation may include aphonia, sore throat, ulcers and granulomas of the larynx and dilation, rupture and stenosis of the trachea.

In spite of these possible complications, correct use of tracheal intubation has become the cornerstone of emergency resuscitation and long- term airway control in the critically ill patient.

Technique of Gastric Intubation

In the conscious patient, gastric intubation usually presents little difficulty, if the patient can assist by swallowing. In all comatose patients, however, gastric intubation may be more difficult. Most comatose patients, particularly CPR cases, should have a nasogastric tube passed, but *after* tracheal intubation. In stupor and coma, it is not advisable to attempt gastric intubation before the airway has been secured with a cuffed tracheal tube, since the gastric tube can provoke vomiting or passive regurgitation and aspiration. The tube renders the esophageal sphincters incompetent. This caveat applies to insertion of both small-bore tubes and large-bore tubes (commonly used for gastric lavage). Furthermore, ventilation-oxygenation and CPR should not be interrupted during gastric intubation.

Insertion of a nasogastric tube in the relaxed comatose patient can be facilitated by use of ample (water-soluble) lubricant. First, insert well-lubricated tube through the nose beyond the «give» of the nasopharyngeal angle. Then, use the other hand to lift the larynx forward to open the upper esophageal sphincter; do this by grasping the larynx from the outside, pressing the thumb on one side and the middle finger on the other side behind the larynx. Now advance the gastric tube to engage into the upper esophagus and feed it into the stomach. If necessary insert your index finger into the hypopharynx for palpation, straightening, and bimanual advancement of the tube. Occasionally a laryngoscope may be helpful so that the tube may be directed into the esophagus under direct vision using Magill's forceps.

Alternatives to Tracheal Intubation

Cricothyroid membrane puncture (cricothyrotomy) and translaryngeal oxygen jet insufflation are two alternative steps of last resort when endotracheal intubation is impossible in an asphyxiating patient and necessary equipment for these alternative techniques is immediately available.

While one operator tries to oxygenate the patient by mask, the other performs cricothyrotomy, which is independent of a supply of oxygen and preferable to translaryngeal jet ventilation in the spontaneously breathing patient. Translaryngeal oxygen jet ventilation, which requires compressed oxygen and the necessary connections for intratracheal insufflation, is preferred over cricothyrotomy as an elective procedure for anesthesia in patients undergoing operations on the upper airway in the presence of laryngeal or supralaryngeal obstruction. In complete obstruction cricothyrotomy should be used, not jet ventilation.

These two alternative measures are rarely needed, but both should be part of the therapeutic repertoire of trained professionals involved in emergency resuscitation.

Cricothyrotomy (Fig. 16). This technique is for spontaneous breathing of air or oxygen, artificial ventilation and suctioning. It requires use of the largest available cannula that does not cause injury to the larynx, i.e., in the adult 6 mm and the large child 3 mm outside diameter. In small children and infants, use a 12 gauge over-the-needle catheter. Merely cutting through the cricothyroid space with a pen knife does not establish an airway. The opening must be kept patent, and a standard adaptor must permit connection of ventilation equipment.

One may teach the «cut-and-poke» cricothyrotomy technique (Safar and Penninckx) shown in Fig. 16, which includes a skin incision and piercing of the membrane under vision. Blind (percutaneous) automatic cricothyrotomy techniques (e.g., with «tracheotome») are hazardous and therefore are not recommended.

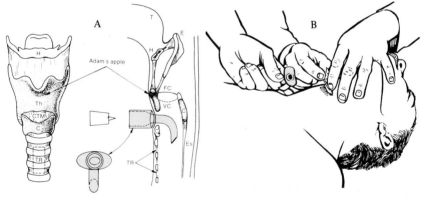

Figure 16: Cricothyrotomy with curved cannula (Safar and Penninckx)
The cannula can be self-made from curved endotracheal tube slip joints (6 mm outside diameter for adults; 3 mm outside diameter for large children), with 15 mm male adaptor to connect ventilation equipment. For small children and infants use 12 gauge over-the-needle catheter.

*(A) **Anatomy with cannula in place.** H, hyoid cartilage; Th, thyroid cartilage; C, cricoid cartilage; TR, trachea; CTM, cricothyroid membrane; E, epiglottis; T, tongue; FC, false cords; VC, vocal cords; Es, esophagus. Bevelled curved cannula. Knife blade with handle (rubber stopper), to be carried safely within 15 mm slip joint of cannula.*

(B) Technique of cricothyrotomy. Place patient supine with head tilted backward. Grasp larynx with thumb and middle finger and identify cricothyroid membrane with index finger. Make adequate horizontal skin incision. Make stab incision through cricothyroid membrane. Poke blunt tip cannula through membrane into tracheal lumen. During IPPV minimize leakage by closing mouth and nose by hand.

Translaryngeal Jet Insufflation (Fig. 17). This technique consists of insertion of a thin over-the-needle catheter through the cricothyroid membrane, with intermittent insufflation of oxygen (Spoerel, Singh, Jacobs, Jacoby, Smith R.). A high pressure source (30−60 psi, 2−4 atmospheres) of oxygen is required to overcome the resistance of the system. The chest must be carefully observed and the valve must be turned off the moment the chest rises to prevent lung rupture.

Passive exhalation is achieved through the upper airway, which must be at least partially open to avoid lung rupture. In cases of complete upper airway obstruction, a second large-bore tracheal catheter needle, perhaps with intermittent suction, should be inserted to accommodate exhalations. Inflation starts with some air entrainment and ends with upward leakage through the larynx. The most life-threatening possible complication (which can be avoided with proper technique) is interstitial oxygen insufflation from lung rupture or from accidental insertion of the catheter into tissue spaces instead of into the tracheal lumen. This tracheal insufflation technique can exsufflate upper airway secretions but does not allow suctioning. For translaryngeal *high frequency* ventilation, see Chapter 1 B (Klain).

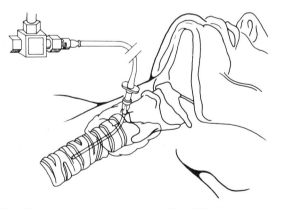

Figure 17: Translaryngeal oxygen jet insufflation
Prepare necessary equipment assembly, consisting of 30−60 psi (2−4 atm) oxygen source, high pressure tubing, valve (three-way

stopcock or push button release valve), extension tubing, and 14—16 gauge over-the-needle catheter.

Hold head tilted backward, hold larynx between thumb and middle finger, and identify cricothyroid membrane with the index finger.

Insert catheter needle through cricothyroid space into tracheal lumen, pointing downward.

Connect extension tube-equipment assembly.

Inflate lungs by turning valve or stopcock until chest moves; then turn valve off and let the patient exhale passively through the mouth and nose.

(From American Heart Association Advanced Life Support Slide Series, 1976).

Other Steps of Airway Control

Tracheotomy, bronchoscopy, bronchodilation and pleural drainage all are elective (though sometimes urgent) procedures, which are adjunctive to the steps of emergency airway control described so far.

Tracheotomy (Fig. 18). It is for long-term airway management and, ideally, should be done under conditions of optimal lighting and sterility in the operating room. In acute emergencies, the skilled operator can perform endotracheal intubation or cricothyroid membrane puncture more rapidly than tracheotomy. (The resulting opening in the tracheal wall is called «tracheostomy»; the opening which results from suturing the entire lumen of the trachea into the skin after laryngectomy is called «tracheostoma»).

A switch from tracheal tube to tracheostomy tube should be considered when tracheal cannulation is expected to be needed longer than 7—10 days, or when the patient is conscious and wishes to talk during prolonged artificial ventilation, which is possible with use of a leaking tracheostomy tube or a «speaking tube», but not an endotracheal (translaryngeal) tube. Whenever possible tracheotomy should be done as an elective procedure and on an oxygenated, well-ventilated patient, if necessary with a tracheal tube in place.

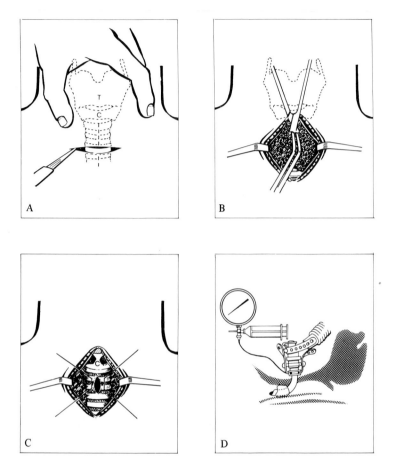

Figure 18: Technique of Tracheotomy

(A) Make horizontal or vertical skin incision.

(B) Ligate and divide the thyroid isthmus if necessary, and expose tracheal rings 1—4.

(C) Ask assistant to withdraw the translaryngeal (endotracheal) tube partially, with the tip remaining in the larynx. Place stay sutures through tracheal rings 2 and 3 on both sides of the anticipated opening, for immediate access to the tracheal lumen in case of tube dislodgement later. Make midline incision of tracheal rings 2 and 3 (oval-shaped or inverted V-shaped excision in adults).

(D) Quickly insert appropriate size tracheostomy tube (Tbl. II A) with large soft cuff. Inflate cuff to abolish audible leak. Connect via nonslip swivel adapter to ventilation-oxygenation device. Remove translaryngeal (endotracheal) tube.

Bronchoscopy.

It is needed to clear the tracheobronchial tree after aspiration of solid foreign matter or obstruction by thick mucus or blood. For tracheobronchial clearing, the rigid tube bronchoscope is more effective than bronchoscopy with the flexible fiberoptic bronchoscope, which has only a narrow lumen for suctioning. Bronchoscopy in critically ill patients (conscious or unconscious) should be undertaken during spontaneous breathing with oxygenation and assisted ventilation, using jet insufflation or a ventilating bronchoscope (Muendnich, Safar). In massive aspiration of solid foreign matter, ventilation bronchoscopy can be a life- saving resuscitative measure.

The flexible fiberoptic bronchoscope (Ikada) has advantages for examination and for removing mucous plugs from smaller bronchi, particularly in the upper lobes. Lung rupture is possible during fiberoptic bronchoscopy through an endotracheal tube with IPPV, if exhalation is impaired by the scope diameter within the tube.

Bronchodilation and clearing. These are important in the management of status asthmaticus, bronchitis with asphyxiation, in near-drowning and in aspiration. Lower airway control should include a combination of: (1) titrated positive pressure ventilation with oxygen (IPPV, CPPV, IPPB or IMV); (2) humidification to promote ciliary escalator clearing; (3) bronchodilation by metaproterenol aerosol plus aminophylline IV; (4) shrinkage of the mucosa by a sympathetic alpha-receptor stimulator aerosol; and (5) arterial pH normalization. Steroid in high doses (e.g., methylprednisolone or dexamethasone) intravenously, or by nonabsorbable steroid aerosol (beclomethasone (betamethasone)) may be essential to control severe asthma. Steroids are not acutely acting bronchodilators, but intravenous steroids begin to help control acute asthma attacks within a few hours (Kampschulte).

Laryngotracheobronchitis may benefit transiently from epinephrine (adrenaline) aerosol administered into the upper airways with assisted or controlled intermittent positive pressure ventilation. *Epiglottitis* with asphyxia, however, calls for endotracheal intubation by an expert, or tracheotomy.

Pleural Drainage (Fig. 19). It is lifesaving in tension pneumothorax, which can asphyxiate the patient rapidly by lung collapse and mediastinal displacement with bronchial kinking and compression, and kinking of the great vessels.

Suspect tension pneumothorax when there is tracheal deviation from the midline on neck palpation, progressive inability of the chest to deflate, deterioration of the pulse, unilateral distension of the chest, distension of the abdomen from inversion of the diaphragm and pneumoperitoneum, tympanism on percussion, mediastinal shift on percussion, and/or interstitial emphysema with subcutaneous crepitation at the neck (from interstitial alveolar rupture). Auscultation can be deceptive.

For emergency pleural drainage, first do a diagnostic tap of the suspected pleural space with a needle in the second intercostal space, mid- clavicular line, in the supine or semi-sitting position. If air escapes, insert a large-bore chest tube and connect it to a one-way valve or drainage system serving the same purpose (Fig. 19). As a temporary measure, several blunt-tip large-bore catheter needles can be inserted. For draining blood or fluid, a chest tube should be inserted just behind the midaxillary line through the 5th or 6th intercostal space. Some use this same posterior (lateral) chest tube with multiple holes, inserted toward the superior anterior aspects of the thoracic cavity, for draining gas at the same time.

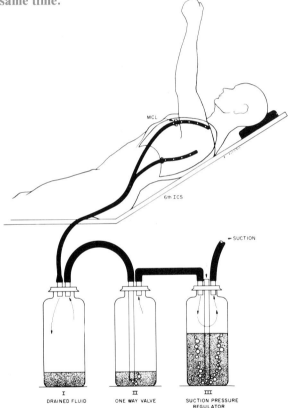

Figure 19: Technique of Pleural Drainage
The appropriate size chest tube is inserted through a stab incision in the skin and into the pleural cavity, with the open technique (blunt Kelly clamp pierced through the intercostal space and pried open for tube insertion) or the closed technique (using trocar).

54

A chest tube with multiple holes is inserted anteriorly through the second intercostal space for draining gas (apical tube); another posteriorly through the fifth or sixth intercostal space just behind the midaxillary line for draining liquid (basal tube). They are connected via a Y-tube to the bottle system consisting of bottle I for collection of fluids; bottle II, a one-way valve; and bottle III to keep a constant controllable negative pressure. For transportation a one-way valve instead of the three bottle system is used. In hospitals the three bottle system may be replaced by new chest suction devices, provided they permit control of negative pressure and a high flow rate.

Chapter I B

BREATHING SUPPORT
Emergency Artificial Ventilation and Oxygenation

Ventilation Patterns (Fig. 20)

Most current methods of artificial ventilation depend on intermittent inflation of the lungs with positive pressure applied to the airway. Thus, intermittent positive pressure (controlled) ventilation (IPPV) is the basic artificial ventilation pattern (Fig. 20A). Research in the 1950s on emergency artificial ventilation without equipment proved the superiority of IPPV with exhaled air over the back-pressure and chest-pressure arm-lift maneuvers then in vogue; the latter techniques in most instances failed to ventilate the lungs, because of inadequate force of inflation and inability of the operator to control the patient's airway (Safar). Therefore, the back-pressure arm-lift (prone) method (Holger-Nielsen), chest-pressure arm-lift (supine) method (Silvester) and other «push-pull» methods of emergency artificial ventilation (Gordon) are obsolete and not recommended anymore.

The forces that must be overcome with IPPV in order to achieve lung inflation are primarily the elastic resistance of the lungs and thorax and the airway resistance. Exhalation is usually passive.

Shallow spontaneous breaths may be augmented with assisted ventilation (patient-triggered, operator- or ventilator-augmented breaths) (Fig. 20A); or with intermittent mandatory ventilation (IMV) (spontaneous breathing with operator- or ventilator-controlled inflations at a superimposed slower rate) (Fig. 20B). All these methods may be performed with exhaled air, air, or oxygen.

During controlled, assisted or intermittent mandatory ventilation, positive end-expiratory pressure (PEEP) is used to open and stabilize (splint) collapsed or fluid-filled alveoli. Expiratory retardation is used to prevent intrapulmonary airway collapse during exhalation in conditions which narrow or soften bronchi (e.g., asthma, emphysema). Negative pressure (PNPV) in the airway is not recommended as it can enhance intrapulmonary airway collapse and pulmonary edema.

Most of the airway pressure patterns of assisted and controlled positive pressure ventilation (Fig. 20) can be provided either without equipment or with only portable equipment, although some would require at least homemade improvisations of customary portable equipment. However, expiratory retardation, PEEP and IMV during artificial ventilation are easier and better performed with use of special mechanical ventilators (Mushin, Safar, Pontoppidan, Petty, Moerch, Kirby, Engstrom).

Prolonged positive pressure ventilation of any kind is better performed via an endotracheal tube or tracheostomy tube. Gastric insufflation frequently occurs when airway pressures exceed 20 cm H_2O. Continuous positive airway pressure (CPAP) of 5 to 15 cm H_2O during spontaneous breathing is possible via mask or mouthpiece; CPAP is provided by inexpensive equipment assembled from available supplies (see oxygen delivery system, below). (Safar, Greenbaum, Gregory).

Lung rupture due to positive airway pressure is related to lung pathology (such as bullous emphysema) and volume of inflation. To deliver adequate tidal volumes, peak airway pressures of 30 cm H_2O or less are usually adequate. Some patients with partial airway obstruction or stiff lungs or chest (low compliance), however, may require 30 to 70 cm H_2O peak pressures. Lung rupture may be prevented by avoiding overdistension, keeping PEEP as low as possible and allowing full passive exhalations. This may require a relatively slow ventilation rate.

Circulatory depression from increased airway pressure and PEEP is related to a high mean intrathoracic pressure and is more likely to occur in patients with normal (compliant) lungs and low blood volume. Patients with stiff lungs who need PEEP are fortunately less likely to develop hypotension, as the stiff lungs «buffer» the transmission of pressure.

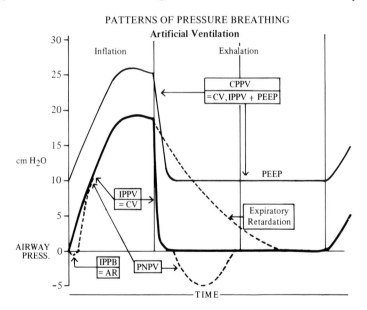

Figure 20: Airway pressure patterns of assisted and controlled positive pressure ventilation.

(A) *IPPV: intermittent positive pressure (controlled) ventilation.*
    CV: controlled ventilation.

Figure 20, (continued)

IPPB: intermittent positive pressure (assisted) breathing.
AR: assisted respiration:
PEEP: positive end-expiratory pressure (for alveolar recruitment).
CPPV: continuous positive pressure ventilation, i.e., IPPV plus PEEP.
*   Expiratory retardation for splinting airways in emphysema.*
PNPV: positive-negative pressure (controlled) ventilation.

Intermittent Mandatory Ventilation

$$IMV = \frac{SB\text{-}Atm.\ P.}{SB\ \text{-}\ CPAP}\ \ \text{or} \quad + \text{IPPV (slow rate)}$$

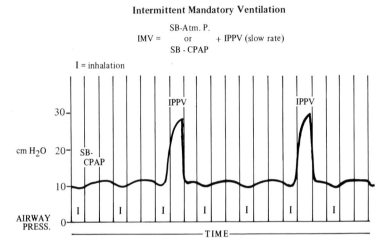

(B) Airway pressure with intermittent mandatory ventilation (IMV), i.e., spontaneous breathing (SB) with continuous positive airway pressure (CPAP), and manual or mechanically controlled lung inflations (IPPV) superimposed (see text). I: spontaneous inhalations. IMV requires a special ventilator.

Direct Mouth-to-Mouth and Mouth-to-Nose Ventilation (Fig. 21)

Exhaled air, which contains 16 to 18 per cent oxygen, has been found to be an adequate resuscitative gas, provided that the patient's lungs are normal and the operator uses about twice normal tidal volumes (Elam). This usually results in arterial PCO_2 values of 20 to 30 mmHg in the rescuer and 30 to 40 mmHg in the patient; and in arterial PO_2 values of over 75 mm Hg (oxygen saturation over 90 per cent) in the patient with normal lungs.

Thus, emergency artificial ventilation should never be delayed by attempts to find and apply adjuncts. Direct exhaled air ventilation is always readily available. In acute apnea, exhaled air immediately does more good than air or oxygen seconds later.

Whenever adequate ventilation (as judged by intermittent chest expansion and escape of exhaled air) cannot be achieved with equipment used for providing IPPV with air or oxygen, immediate return to mouth-to-mouth ventilation is indicated.

Sequence for direct exhaled air ventilation (Fig. 21).
1 It the patient is unconscious, tilt his/her head backward.
2 If he is not breathing, inflate his lungs by blowing into his mouth.
3 If this meets an obstruction, close his mouth and blow into his nose.
4 If this is also unsuccessful, make sure his head is tilted backward, displace his mandible forward, retract his lower lip, and try once again to blow into his mouth (using the triple airway maneuver).

Technique of mouth-to-mouth ventilation (Fig. 21 A).
1 Tilt the patient's head backward, with one hand on his forehead and the other under his neck.

2 If his mouth is closed or chin is sagging, move your hand from under the neck to support his chin and to hold his mouth slightly open.

3 Take a deep breath, seal your mouth around the patient's mouth (mouth and nose in infants and small children) with a wide open circle, and blow forcefully into adults, gently into children (use only puffs for infants to avoid lung rupture). When blowing into the mouth, prevent air leakage through his nose, either by pinching it with one hand or by pressing your cheek against the nostrils while blowing. While blowing, watch his chest to see whether it rises with your inflation.

4 When you see the patient's chest rise, stop inflation; release the seal of your mouth against the patient's mouth; turn your face to the side; and allow the patient to exhale passively.

5 When his exhalation is finished, give him the next deep inflation. Volume is more important than rhythm. Repeat inflations in adults about every 5 seconds (12 per minute); in children about every 3 seconds (20 per minute).

The process of blowing air into the patient's mouth not only inflates the lungs but may also force air into the *stomach,* particularly when the air passage is obstructed or the inflation pressure excessive. Inflation of the stomach may make lung inflations more difficult and provoke regurgitation and aspiration. Therefore, if the patient's stomach bulges markedly, to the extent that it interferes with ventilation, press with your hand briefly over the epigastrium (between sternum and umbilicus). This will force air out of the stomach. Since this maneuver may also cause regurgitation, tilt the patient's head down if possible, and turn the head and shoulders to one side and be prepared to clear his pharynx. As soon as possible after suspected aspiration, intubate and suction the trachea, and drain the stomach via a naso-gastric tube.

Technique of mouth-to-nose ventilation (Fig. 21 B).

When blowing into the mouth meets obstruction, (or when the mouth is not easily accessible as with resuscitation started in water), switch to mouth-to-nose ventilation. This also is necessary when it is impossible to open the patient's mouth (trismus), as during seizures (convulsions).

1 Cup one hand under the patient's chin and close his mouth with your thumb.
2 Take a deep breath; encircle the patient's nose with your mouth (avoid pinching his nose with your lips); and blow. Open his mouth during exhalation, as he may have expiratory naso-pharyngeal obstruction.

In most countries mouth-to-mouth ventilation is taught as first step, with mouth-to-nose as an alternative. In some countries, mouth-to-nose is the preferred method. Both methods should be taught to all personnel.

The *sequence* of Steps A, B, C, — after having established unresponsiveness:

The start to ventilation-oxygenation fits into the entire CPR sequence as follows:

1 Apply 3 to 5 rapid, deep lung inflations.
2 Feel for the pulse.
3 If the pulse is present, continue with one inflation every 5 seconds (about 12 inflations per minute). In children, a rate of one inflation about every 3 seconds (about 20 inflations per minute) is desirable.
4 If the pulse is absent, start external cardiac compressions and proceed with CPR (Step C).

Ensure adequate ventilation by observing the patient's chest to determine whether it rises and falls, feeling air moving from you into him, and hearing and feeling air escape during exhalations.

Some individuals may find it easier to overcome their hesitations regarding direct mouth-to-mouth contact for exhaled air ventilation by blowing through a *handkerchief* placed over the patient's mouth and nose.

In unconscious victims of *trauma,* for spontaneous and/or mouth-to-mouth breathing, gently tilt the head backward only moderately (not maximally), apply gentle axial traction and, if necessary, displace the mandible forward. Flexion (chin on chest) and lateral turning of the head and neck must be avoided in patients with suspected neck injury. Nevertheless, the airway must have precedence over other priorities.

In the *tracheotomized* patient or *laryngectomee,* perform direct mouth-to-tracheostomy tube, or mouth-to-stoma inflations. Improvise control of leaks between tube and skin.

In *small children and infants,* exhaled air ventilation is performed with the same technique, except that the rescuer covers both the mouth and nose

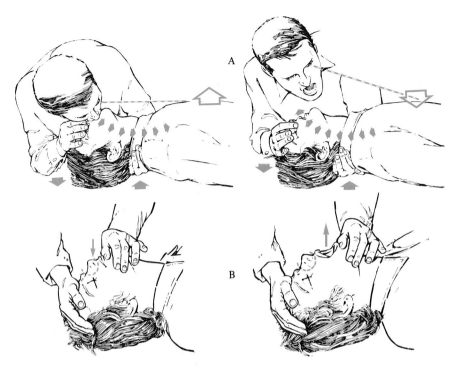

Figure 21: Exhaled air ventilation.

(A) Mouth-to moutn (with head tilt by neck lift)
(B) Mouth-to-nose (with head tilt by chin support). Inflation (left) and passive exhalation (right).

of the child with his mouth and uses small breaths of less volume to inflate the lungs at a more rapid rate, about once every 2 seconds. In newborn babies, the volume between your cheeks is adequate, i.e., ventilate with «puffs». Backward tilt of the head should not be exaggerated, since the infant's flexible hyperextended cervical spine may worsen the obstruction.

Mouth-to-Adjunct Ventilation (Fig. 11C, 22)
Since the development of mouth-to-mouth ventilation, the first adjuncts recommended for exhaled air ventilation were a mask (Elam) and the S-tube (Safar). These devices were suggested in order to make the introduction of mouth-to-mouth ventilation more acceptable when people objected on hygienic grounds. Experience since the 1950s has shown that in emergencies, lay people rarely hesitate to apply oral resuscitation directly, and that adjuncts are usually not immediately available. Therefore, the lay public should not be taught mouth-to-mouth with the use of tubes or masks in preference to the direct mouth-to-mouth method.

Mouth-to-airway (Fig. 11C). The S-tube (Safar), a double Guedel airway overcomes the esthetic objection to direct mouth-to-mouth contact, keeps the victim's mouth open, and assists in maintaining a patent airway. Like all pharyngeal tubes, however, it may induce gagging, laryngospasm or vomiting, if inserted into the conscious or merely stuporous patient. Shortened S-tubes or mouth props obviate upper airway stimulation, but may cause problems with air leakage and obstruction. The Brooke Airway is a modified S-tube incorporating a separate exhalation valve. Hospital and ambulance personnel have used S-tubes and regular pharyngeal tubes effectively. For details see pages 30 — 32.

Mouth-to-mask with oxygen (Fig. 22). The Laerdal pocket mask can be used safely by trained lay personnel, but does not improve ventilation efficacy over direct mouth-to-mouth (Breivik, Esposito). The main advantage of the pocket (folding) mask is its oxygen nipple for delivery of 50 to 100 per cent oxygen, depending on the oxygen flow (Safar).

All types of trained personnel attempting to ventilate manikins and patients seem to be more effective with the mouth-to-mask than with the bag-valve-mask technique. The latter leaves only one hand free for support of mask fit and head tilt (which closes the mouth under the mask), does not usually permit jaw thrust during IPPV by one operator, and often provides less than 1 liter inflation volume, which is hardly enough to overcome the leakage with a poor mask fit. In contrast, the Laerdal pocket mask provides up to 4 liters reserve volume (the rescuer's vital capacity) to overcome leakage, and keeps both hands free for mask fit and jaw thrust. When jaw thrust is required, mouth-to-mask ventilation is more easily performed than mouth-to-mouth, since the operator can remain positioned at the patient's vertex. The Laerdal pocket mask with oxygen nipple provides an inspired oxygen concentration of 50 to 80 per cent during spontaneous breathing and 50 to 100 per cent during artificial ventilation with delivered flow rates of 15 liters per minute.

Masks should be transparent to permit recognition of cyanosis, vomitus, mucus and blood, and clouding with spontaneous exhalations for monitoring. There should be an effectively sealing cuff, oxygen insufflation nipple, breathing port with a standard 15/22 mm connector, and a head strap to loosely hold the mask to the patient's face during spontaneous breathing and one operator CPR, when continuous holding of the mask is not possible. The masks should fit adults, children and infants. The Laerdal pocket mask fits all ages; for infants it covers the entire face and should be applied upside down, with the nose part of the mask over the chin.

Recent studies in Norway and the USA indicate that use of the pocket mask helps lay persons to learn the technique of exhaled air ventilation on each other without manikins, and encourages learning to displace the mandible forward (jaw thrust). The latter is particularly desirable for use in accident victims in lieu of maximal backward tilt of the head.

A

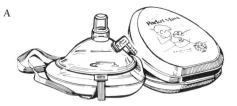

Figure 22: Pocket mask with oxygen insufflation nipple for mouth-to-mask ventilation with oxygen and spontaneous inhalation of oxygen (Safar: Crit Care Med 2:273, 1974).

(A) Laerdal pocket transparent folding mask with 15 mm male breathing port and oxygen insufflation nipple, inflated cushion, and head strap.

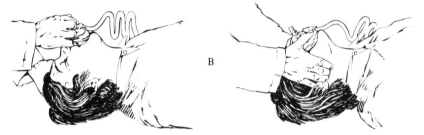

B

(B) In comatose patient, tilt head backward. Open mouth by retracting lower lip and apply rim of mask over chin to keep mouth open. Apply entire mask over mouth and nose.

C

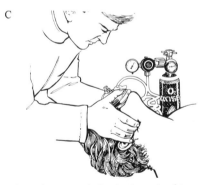

(C) Clamp mask to face, with both thumbs (thenar eminences) on top of mask and fingers 2 to 5 of both hands grasping both ascending rami of mandible in front of earlobes. Pull forcefully upward (forward) so that lower teeth are in front of upper teeth and chin juts out. Mouth should remain open under mask. Front of neck must be maximally stretched. Do not pull on chin, as this tends to close mouth. Take a deep breath, blow into mask until chest moves, take mouth off, and let him exhale passively.

Sustain this maneuver as long as the patient is unconscious or until a pharyngeal or endotracheal tube can be inserted. For long-term ventilation a pharyngeal tube is helpful, as it can usually replace jaw thrust.

In infants apply mask upside down and cover the entire face. In infants use only puffs from your cheeks.

When oxygen is available, deliver it via the nipple of the mask. Oxygen at 10 to 15 liters per minute continuous flow results in about 50 per cent oxygen inhaled. With higher flows, artificial ventilation with 100 per cent oxygen is possible by intermittently occluding the breathing port with your tongue, and opening it when the chest rises to permit exhalation.

For use during CPR or in the spontaneously breathing patient, when continuous manual support of mask fit is not possible, strap the mask to the face loosely.

Bag-Valve-Mask with Oxygen (Fig. 23)

The development of the self-refilling bag-valve-mask unit (Ruben) followed the bellows-valve-mask devices of the Oxford and Kreiselman types, used during World War II. Ruben's unit is made by Ambu.

Obtaining a tight seal at the mask proved difficult with the bellows device — there was a tendency to push the chin down and obstruct the airway when the bellows was squeezed, and the operator could not feel the resistance encountered.

The self-refilling bag-valve unit is not easy to use in the nonintubated patient (ventilation by mask), but is particularly valuable and effective for ventilation and oxygenation of the intubated patient, which can easily be mastered by nonphysicians. Its 1 to 1.5 liter size bag provides less reserve gas volume in case of leakage than does mouth-mask-oxygen, and does not leave both hands free to provide jaw thrust. Therefore, the operator must be prepared to insert a pharyngeal tube and must be experienced with and skillful in the use of these devices.

The bag-valve-mask permits delivery of oxygen during both spontaneous and artificial ventilation (Fig. 23A). It should consist of a self-refilling bag with an inlet valve to which an oxygen reservoir tube (Fig. 23B) or reservoir bag (Fig. 23C) may be attached, and a non-rebreathing valve at the mask or tracheal tube. In order to deliver 100 per cent oxygen, the reservoir must be at least as large as the tidal volume (bag volume) and the oxygen inflow rate must at least equal the minute volume. The non-rebreathing valve must have an expiratory valve to permit delivery of the gas mixture from the bag during spontaneous breathing. The device should be easy to clean and disinfect and have a non-sticking valve that does not permit backward leak, and that does not lock in the inflation position during delivery of oxygen. There should be transparent, well-fitting face masks of various sizes; and valve connections with a 22 mm male fitting to the mask and 15 mm female fitting to tracheal tubes and other devices. It should be impossible to assemble the components of the bag-valve-mask unit incorrectly. Although the main advantage of the bag-valve-mask unit constructed as described above is its ability to deliver 100 per cent oxygen, in some examples an excessive oxygen flow rate with slow bag release may cause the valve to lock in the inspiratory position and cause lung rupture. For the same reason oxygen must never be delivered under pressure directly into the self-refilling bag.

Among the commercially available units, the Laerdal RFB II unit fulfills the above requirements best (Fig. 23) (Nobel, Safar and Lind).

Since use of the bag-valve-mask unit usually closes the mouth under the mask, some unconscious patients require an oropharyngeal or nasopharyngeal tube to overcome nasal obstruction.

The *technique* is as follows (Fig 23):
1 Position yourself at the patient's vertex. Tilt his head backward. If he is relaxed, insert an oropharyngeal or nasopharyngeal tube.

2 Spread the mask, mold it over the patient's mouth and nose, clamp it to his face with one hand, tilt his head backward, and squeeze the bag until the chest rises.

3 Release the bag for exhalation. Abrupt bag release is necessary for proper valve function.

For *clamping the mask* to the patient's face use one of the following two maneuvers:
1 Press with your thumb over the nose part of the mask and with the index finger over the chin part, and use your middle, ring and little fingers to pull the chin upward and backward (Fig. 23B, C).

2 With a flat mask, hook your fingers around the patient's chin and apply pressure on the top of the mask with the palm of your hand, always maintaining backward tilt (Fig. 23D).

With an oxygen flow of over 10 liters per minute, the inhaled oxygen concentration in adults is 80 to 100% when using a reservoir; and 30 to 50% without reservoir.

Holding mask and head with one hand and providing additional jaw thrust is difficult for the inexperienced. You may use your knee or hip, for reinforcing head-tilt and your chin for reinforcing mask fit.

If you must use both hands for providing mask fit and jaw thrust, ask your assistant to squeeze the bag. You also can squeeze the bag between your arm (elbow) and your waist, if you use an extension tube between nonrebreathing valve and bag.

Modifications of the self-refilling bag-valve-mask unit permit special uses:

(1) Anesthesia with minimal equipment for field conditions (Pearson).

(2) Bronchodilator aerosol administration, with a nebulizer interposed

between non-rebreathing valve and patient (Milai).

(3) IPPV with 100 per cent oxygen plus adjustable PEEP, with a modified Laerdal unit (Fig. 23E) (Safar and Lind). This may be lifesaving in pulmonary edema, aspiration, near-drowning, or other conditions associated with increased pulmonary shunting.

Spontaneous breathing with continuous positive airway pressure (SB-CPAP) reqires a special equipment assembly (see first and last sections of this chapter). Most self-refilling bag-valve-mask units can not be used safely for SB-CPAP, as sustained positive pressure can lock the non-rebreathing valve in the inflation position and cause lung rupture.

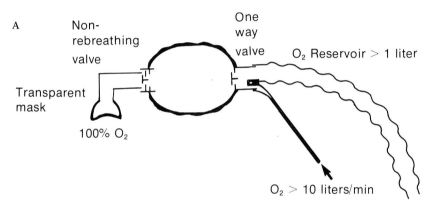

Figure 23: Self-refilling bag-valve-mask unit with oxygen
(A) Diagram of self-refilling bag with inlet valve, oxygen tube reservoir, and non-rebreathing valve.

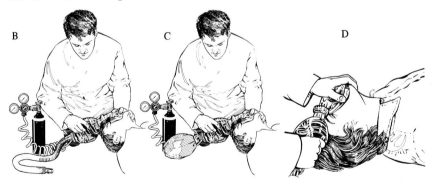

(B) Laerdal Resusci-Folding Bag II with large-bore tube oxygen reservoir.

(C) Laerdal Resusci-Folding Bag II with bag oxygen reservoir (with safety inlet and overflow valves).

A continuous flow of oxygen is delivered into the reservoir at atmospheric pressure.

Clamping the mask to the patient's face with regular grip (B & C); or an improved method (D) with fingers pulling on chin and palm of hand pressing mask downward.

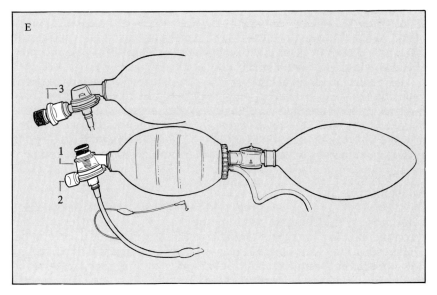

(E) Bag-valve-tube unit (Laerdal) for IPPV with PEEP and 100 % O₂.

(1) Combined PEEP/Non-rebreathing Valve (Laerdal) with Expiration Diverter (2).

(3) Separate PEEP valve (Ambu) mounted on the expiration port of a standard Laerdal Non-rebreathing Valve.

Manually-Triggered Oxygen-Powered Ventilators

Oxygen-powered manually-triggered ventilation devices (e.g., Elder valve, Robertshaw valve) permit instantaneous manual initiation and termination of positive pressure inflation with oxygen. These units are recommended:

(a) If they can deliver 100 per cent oxygen;

(b) Provide instantaneous flow rates of 1 liter per second or more for adults (with lower adjustable flow rates for infants and children);

(c) Have the manual trigger positioned so that both hands of the operator can remain at the mask to provide jaw thrust while triggering inflation;

(d) Have a safety valve to pop off at about 50 cm H_2O for adults (with a switch to 30 cm H_2O for infants and children);

(e) Have standard 15 mm female/22 mm male fittings; and

(f) Function as a demand oxygen inhalation device for spontaneous breathing.

The demand valve (inhalator) should be highly sensitive so that flow rates follow the patient's demand without excessive airway pressure fluctuations, even during tachypnea.

High instantaneous flow rates have been recommended for CPR to enable interposition of ventilations between chest compressions. These high flow rates, however, may cause high pharyngeal pressures and gastric distention. Therefore, such devices which provide high flow rates are more effective when used with a tracheal tube.

The principal disadvantages of oxygen-powered manually-triggered ventilation devices, in comparison with the bag-valve-mask and mouth- to-mask techniques, are their dependence on compressed gas; the inability of the operator to feel resistance during inflation; unchecked peak inflation pressure able to cause gastric insufflation, regurgitation, lung rupture and tension pneumothorax; inability to deliver humidified oxygen; and need for additional training.

Automatic Ventilators

Most old-style *oxygen-powered* automatically cycling *fixed-pressure* ventilators (resuscitators) used in the past in ambulances are not recommended for emergency artificial ventilation without tracheal tube. The reasons that such devices are not in favor is that the fixed cycling pressure does not permit adaptation of inflation volume, pressure, flow and rhythm to the changing mask leakage, lung-thorax compliance, airway resistance and spontaneous breathing efforts. The «suck-and-blow» units in addition interfere with passive exhalation. During external chest compressions, because of inadequate pressure and flow rate, these devices tend to cycle prematurely into exhalation. Their heavy weight, complexity, and cost are added disadvantages and many of them cannot be adapted for a continuous flow if required.

Some new *adjustable-pressure* oxygen-powered automatic ventilators, such as the Bird Mark VII are exceptions. Some are small and portable, and can provide many of the ventilation patterns shown in figure 20. They have been used successfully for ventilating intubated patients with near-normal lungs, not only in hospitals but also in ambulances.

For prolonged mechanical ventilation of the intubated patient with abnormal lungs, in the hospital, a great variety of suitable automatic ventilators with adjustable and readable airway pressure, tidal volume, flow rates and cycling rate could be recommended. These ventilators should be capable of producing IPPV with or without PEEP, and intermittent mandatory ventilation or assisted ventilation — with controllable inhaled oxygen concentrations and capability of delivering drug aerosols and warm humidity. *Volume-set,* time cycled ventilators are preferred.

Most *motor powered* mechanical ventilators, favored in intensive care units because of their reliability, are not suitable for emergency artificial ventilation or long-term ventilation in ambulances, as they are not portable and depend on electric line current.

The *tank ventilator* (body box, iron lung), one of the earliest mechanical ventilators, is *not* recommended, not even for prolonged ventilation, as it provides inadequate ventilation power, adjustability and airway control, and makes the patient inaccessible and immobile (Ibsen, Safar). It ventilates by intermittent negative pressure around the body, with the airway exposed to atmospheric pressure.

Translaryngeal oxygen jet ventilation (Chapter 1 A, page 50, Fig. 17) is ready for clinical trials in emergency resuscitation. Its basic mode is with regular ventilation rates. Although an invasive method, it may simplify emergency ventilation and oxygenation in the hands of specially trained personnel.

High frequency ventilation with 100 per cent oxygen (Klain) challenges established concepts of physiologic dead space and alveolar ventilation. There are three modes developed in the laboratory and presently under clinical trial:

(1) High frequency IPPV with rates up to 100 per minute, via tracheal tube (Sjøstrand). Estimated tidal volumes are near or greater than dead space.

(2) High frequency jet ventilation via small gauge catheter inserted into the trachea percutaneously (via cricothyroid membrane or via tracheal or tracheostomy tube), with frequencies of 100 to 500 per minute and tidal volumes smaller than dead space (Klain).

(3) High frequency oscillations with frequencies of 500 to 3000 per minute via open, valveless tracheal tube (Lunkenheimer).

These high cycling rates are produced by portable jet ventilators with fluidic or electric valves. They produce mean airway pressures of 5 to 7 cm H_2O, provided the upper airway is open. High frequency ventilation in the absence of «adequate tidal volumes» can maintain arterial PO_2 and PCO_2 values normal during apnea, perhaps through gas channeling or vibration (oscillation) — enhanced diffusion.

Advantages include low airway pressure (less pulmonary barotrauma), no need for synchronization with spontaneous breathing, and, when used with translaryngeal catheter, less injury to the tracheal mucosa and counteracting aspiration and soft tissue obstruction. Possible disadvantages include inability to suction the tracheobronchial tree, percutaneous cannulation, risk of tissue insufflation, dependence on special equipment, and requirement of an at least partially open upper airway for exhalations. The ability of high frequency ventilation to reverse pulmonary shunting (recruit alveoli) in pulmonary edema and consolidation (ARDS) has not yet been documented.

Oxygen Delivery Systems (Fig. 24)

During emergency resuscitation, additional oxygen should be introduced as soon as it becomes available, in order to increase the margin of safety in oxygen delivery. While healthy lungs permit full oxygenation of arterial blood with use of exhaled air or air, most patients requiring resuscitation have abnormal lungs. This includes some alveoli, unventilated because of being collapsed or fluid-filled, and others less ventilated than perfused. Thus optimal resuscitation requires a higher inspired oxygen concentration than that provided in exhaled air or air.

For emergency resuscitation, use 100 per cent oxygen first if available. Inhalation of 100 per cent oxygen is safe for at least 6 hours, but the concentration should be reduced within about 6 to 12 hours if arterial PO_2 permits, to about 50 per cent, to avoid pulmonary destruction by oxygen. This occurs at about 48 hours of 100 per cent oxygen inhalation (Comroe). Fifty per cent oxygen appears to be safe for unlimited long-term use. However, sick lungs (shunting) increase tolerance of greater than 50 % O_2 inhaled (Winter).

Oxygen administration by any method requires an oxygen source, such as a portable small cylinder; a moveable large oxygen cylinder as found on emergency vehicles and in hospitals; or piped wall oxygen (Fig. 24). Appropriate yoke, valve, flowmeter, humidifier, and connecting tubing to the patient's oxygen administration equipment are as important as the oxygen cylinder and the mask. This equipment must be understood by all health care personnel involved in resuscitation and intensive care. Oxygen sources must be capable of delivering oxygen at 30 to 60 pounds per square inch pressure (about 2 to 4 atmospheres) to resuscitators and mechanical ventilators; and be available to deliver oxygen at near atmospheric pressure at controllable flow rates for mask and bag-valve units. For emergency resuscitation, exact oxygen concentrations are not necessary. For evaluation of arterial PO_2 values, however, and for long- term respiratory care, knowing the exact oxygen concentration inhaled is desirable. This requires control over the oxygen concentration delivered, which is facilitated with use of air/oxygen mixers, and a leak-free system.

Dry air or oxygen inhaled for prolonged periods stops pulmonary clearing and promotes pulmonary infection. Adequate natural humidification is only possible when breathing through the nose. For long-term oxygen inhalation through the mouth, endotracheal tube or tracheostomy tube, the oxygen must be humidified and ideally also warmed to about body temperature. Cold bubble humidifiers are inadequate for long-term use. Warmed bubble or surface humidifiers are preferred over nebulizers, since the latter offer a greater risk of droplet-mediated iatrogenic infection.

Recommended for emergency resuscitation cases with spontaneous breathing is oxygen administration via the simple versatile Laerdal pocket folding mask (Fig. 22), or the self-refilling bag-valve-mask unit (Fig. 23).

For spontaneous breathing of humidified oxygen via tracheal tube, the patient is best connected to a large-bore valveless T-tube (with short tail). Customary flow rates (e.g., 10 liters per minute) will provide inhaled oxygen concentrations lower than those delivered bacause air is inhaled as well. Inhaled oxygen concentrations, however, will equal delivered concentrations with use of the T-tube when inflow rates exceed average peak inspiratory flow rates (approx. 20 to 25 liters per minute in the adult). Artificial ventilation is possible by intermittently occluding the tail of the T-tube. The chest must be watched to prevent lung rupture.

During spontaneous breathing (SB) of 50 to 100 per cent oxygen (via strapped-on mask, mouth piece or tracheal tube), arterial PO_2 can often be raised further in the presence of reversible shunting (e.g., pulmonary edema) by adding *continuous positive airway pressure* (SB-CPAP) of 5 to 15 cm H_2O. This can be provided with equipment assembled from available components (see Safar and Caroline: Chapter 10 in Schwartz G, et al., Principles and Practice of Emergency Medicine, Philadelphia, Saunders publ., 1978). This technique is not essential for CPR, but represents a useful

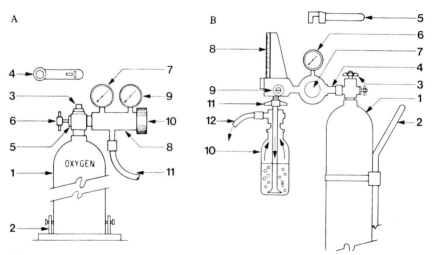

Figure 24:

(A). **Portable oxygen delivery system.** *(1) Small cylinder, (2) stand, (3) cylinder valve, (4) wrench, (5) yoke, (6) yoke handle, (7) cylinder pressure gauge, (8) reducing valve, (9) flow meter, (10) needle valve, and (11) delivery tube.*

(B). **Moveable oxygen delivery system.** *(1) Large cylinder, (2) moveable cart, (3) cylinder valve, (4) yoke, (5) wrench for fastening yoke, (6) cylinder pressure gauge, (7) reducing valve, (8) flow meter, (9) needle valve, (10) bubble humidifier, (11) wing nut for humidifier, and (12) delivery tube.*

addition to advanced respiratory care (Gregory; Greenbaum).

Not recommended for emergency resuscitation cases are the oxygen delivery systems commonly used for conscious patients, e.g., semi-open valveless oronasal masks with or without bags; the aerosol oxygen mask; the nasal cannula; the nasopharyngeal oxygen catheter (obsolete); the oxygen tent and the Venturi mask.

The Venturi mask is a semi-open oronasal mask delivering known inhaled oxygen concentrations of 24 to 40 per cent. It is recommended for stable chronic obstructive pulmonary disease patients without shunting who may hypoventilate when given higher concentrations of oxygen to breathe. If acutely decompensated or in need of resuscitation, these patients should be given higher concentrations of oxygen, but their ventilation assisted or controlled, or spontaneous breathing continuously verbally coached.

Selecting Ventilation and Oxygenation Techniques (Table III)
Emergency resuscitation should begin with hyperventilation by IPPV, using 100 per cent oxygen if available. After re-oxygenation, tidal volume and rate requirements vary greatly between patients and disease states. Proof of the adequacy of *alveolar ventilation* is an arterial PCO_2 of 35 to 45 mm Hg; and proof of the adequacy of *oxygenation* is an arterial PO_2 of at least 80 mm Hg. The acid-base status is reflected in arterial pH and base excess (see Chapter II, Fig. 35).

Arterial blood gas determinations are usually not available during emergency artificial ventilation and not available at all in poorly equipped hospitals. Where arterial blood gas determinations are not available, clinical judgment should be used to suspect hypercarbia (somnolence, poor chest movements) and hypoxemia (restlessness, tachycardia, cyanosis). Absence of cyanosis does not rule out hypoxemia. When in doubt, give oxygen and assist or control ventilation.

For post-resuscitative intensive care, arterial punctures or catheterization for blood gas determinations are highly desirable. The required skills and equipment should be provided in every emergency hospital.

When, after cardiac arrest and restoration of spontaneous circulation, the patient resumes spontaneous breathing, it is desirable to continue controlled ventilation with 50 to 100 per cent oxygen as long as he is unconscious. When he recovers consciousness, inhalation of oxygen should be continued at least until hospital admission, when his care will be assumed by personnel experienced in advanced respiratory therapy and further adjustments made. Even if the patient did not receive CPR and is breathing spontaneously, he should if he is cyanotic or dyspneic also inhale 50 to 100 per cent oxygen during transportation.

For *controlled ventilation* of the comatose patient in the absence of blood gas determinations, ventilate with 50 per cent oxygen, using tidal volumes of approximately 15 ml/kg body weight (1000 ml/70 kg), approximately 12 times per minute (1 inflation every 5 seconds). In the absence of lung changes this will maintain arterial PCO_2 at 25 to 35 mmHg and arterial PO_2 over 100 mmHg in most cases.

Subsequent adjustment of artificial ventilation must take into account at least the following: (1) peak inspiratory airway pressure; (2) tidal volume; (3) rate; and (4) inhaled oxygen concentration. Additional considerations include PEEP, inspiratory flow rate and expiratory flow rate.

Most patients with near-normal lungs can be ventilated adequately with any simple, inexpensive ventilator. Patients with abnormal lungs may require expensive volume-set ventilators with multiple adjustments; if such apparatus is not available, manual IPPV with bag-valve unit or an anesthesia circuit can provide most of the patterns shown in Fig. 20, pg. 57.

Oxygenation of arterial blood will require one or more of the following measures:

1 Provision of ventilation volumes and rates adequate to keep arterial PCO_2 at normal or low levels.
2 Increase of inhaled oxygen to about 50 per cent. If the lungs are healthy, exhaled air or air is adequate. However, augmentation of inspired oxygen concentration to about 50 per cent is needed when some lung areas are relatively less ventilated than perfused.
3 Increase of inhaled oxygen to 50 to 100 per cent and addition of some form of continuous positive pressure for alveolar recruitment. This is needed when there is alveolar shunting (some blood flowing through nonventilated alveoli).
4 Optimization of cardiac output (blood volume and pressure, and heart pumping action). Low cardiac output in the presence of shunting reduces arterial PO_2.

Arterial oxygen transport to the organism is blood flow (cardiac output) times arterial oxygen content. Arterial oxygen transport not only requires an adequate arterial PO_2, but also an adequate blood hemoglobin concentration (hematocrit of 30 to 40 %) and adequate blood flow (which in turn requires adequate blood volume, arterial pressure and cardiac pumping action).

For failure of ventilation, a systematic progression of measures from spontaneous via assisted to controlled ventilation is recommended (Table III A). For failure of oxygenation, a stepwise increase in the complexity of positive pressure techniques and other measures is recommended (Table III B). The objective of these measures will be to maintain near-normal levels of arterial PCO_2, PO_2 and pH.

To guide oxygenation therapies, changes in arterial PO_2 during inhalation of a known oxygen concentration should be observed (alveolar-

TABLE III

Stepwise selection of ventilation patterns
(see Fig. 20)

(A)

Failure of Ventilation
(Airway, muscle or CNS Dysfunction)

Indications: $PaCO_2 > 45$ mmHg
Inspir. capacity ("sigh") < 15 ml/kg body weight

Treatment: Use FIO_2 30 − 50% . . . . Airway press. at
end-exhalation is
Steps   0−5 cm H_2O
for steps (1)−(4)
(1) Spontaneous breathing
(2) Assisted ventilation or IMV
(3) IPPV (Controlled ventilation)
(4) IPPV with expiratory retardation to minimize wheezing

(B)

Failure of Oxygenation
(Alveolar Dysfunction)

Indications: $PaO_2 < 100$ mmHg (FIO_2 50%)

Treatment: Use FIO_2 50 − 100% . . . . Airway press. at
(100% less than 6 hours)   end-exhalation is
5 − > 20 cm H_2O (titrated)
Steps   for steps (1)−(5)
(1) Spontaneous breathing
(2) Spontaneous breathing with CPAP
(3) IMV
(4) IPPV without PEEP
with low PEEP 5 − 10 cm H_2O
with high PEEP 10 − 20 cm H_2O
with "Super PEEP" greater than 20 cm H_2O
(5) Improve circulation, metabolism, colloid osmotic
pressure, osmolality, fluids, electrolytes, renal function
(diuretic, dialysis)

For weaning, use sequence of steps in reverse.

For abbreviations, see glossary.

arterial PO_2 gradient). With art. PO_2 values, list inhaled O_2% (FIO_2).

The *100 per cent oxygen test,* recommended for guiding the therapies of Table IIIB, is carried out as follows:

Test 1 — Determine the arterial PO_2 during breathing of air at atmospheric pressure for at least 5 minutes (this step should be omitted when the patient requires oxygen, which is usually the case during emergency resuscitation). If arterial PO_2 is less than 80 mm Hg, go to test 2.

Test 2 — Determine the arterial PO_2 after at least 5 minutes of 100 per cent oxygen breathing at atmospheric pressure (spontaneous breathing), for instance by bag-valve-mask unit. With normal lungs the arterial PO_2 should be 500 to 600 mm Hg. If arterial PO_2 is 100 mm Hg, a 20 per cent shunt is estimated; if 50 mm Hg, a 50 per cent shunt. Precise determination of shunt is complicated and usually not necessary. If arterial PO_2 is less than about 200 mmHg, go to test 3.

Test 3 — Determine the arterial PO_2 after at least 5 minutes of some form of positive pressure ventilation with 100 per cent oxygen. This reveals whether the shunting found in test 2 is partially reversible by positive airway pressure, and which form of therapy is most effective. Bring the arterial PO_2 to at least 60 mm Hg in the conscious patient, or at least 100 mm Hg in the unconscious patient, by following the steps of Table III B.

During controlled ventilation, PEEP can be optimized by monitoring changes in central venous PO_2, which would drop below about 35 mm Hg when blood flow is reduced by excessive PEEP. Optimizing PEEP is also possible by monitoring airway pressure fluctuations required for a given tidal volume (compliance); the pressure should be minimized (compliance optimized) (Suter).

When the patient recovers consciousness, weaning from controlled via intermittent mandatory (or assisted) ventilation to spontaneous breathing should be with oxygen enrichment. Weaning should be guided not only by blood gas values and clinical measurements but also by clinical judgement, common sense and the patient's ability to cooperate.

Safe indications and techniques for *oxygen administration* in abnormal pressure conditions need special physiologic knowledge and logistic considerations. These conditions include *high altitude* (Safar) and *hyperbarism* (diving, high pressure chamber) (Winter). *Hyperbaric oxygen* needs re-investigation for use in prolonged resuscitation.

Important: Successful resuscitation requires more than ventilation and oxygenation. Oxygen and substrate delivery to tissues depends on tissue perfusion and arterial oxygen content. Tissue perfusion depends on cardiac output, which in turn is governed by venous return, cardiac pumping action and peripheral resistance. Arterial oxygen content depends on the arterial PO_2 and hemoglobin content. Blood flow equals pressure gradient divided by resistance. Peripheral resistance varies between and within different vascular beds; it is increased where there is vasospasm, tissue edema, blood sludging or clotting. Thus, the measures described in Chapters IC, II and III are important for tissue oxygenation.

Chapter I C

Cardiac Resuscitation

Causes of Cardiac Arrest

Cardiac arrest may be primary or secondary. The most common cause of *primary* cardiac arrest is ventricular fibrillation from (transient) inhomogeneous myocardial ischemia. Other causes of primary arrest include ventricular fibrillation and asystole from heart disease, electric shock or drugs.

Secondary cardiac arrest can develop rapidly or slowly, and is most commonly caused by asphyxia or exsanguination. Examples of *rapid* secondary cardiac arrest include alveolar anoxia (from pulmonary edema or inhalation of oxygen-free gas), asphyxia from airway obstruction or apnea, and rapid blood loss. Examples of *slow* secondary cardiac arrest include severe hypoxemia (from pneumonia or pulmonary edema-consolidation, i.e., shock lung); cardiogenic, oligemic or distributive (septic) type shock; and acute brain insults (leading to medullary failure and severe intractable hypotension and apnea).

Sudden complete cessation of circulation, from whatever cause, results in unconsciousness within about 15 seconds; an isoelectric EEG in 15 to 30 seconds: agonal gasping for 30 to 60 seconds; and apnea and maximal pupillary dilatation starting at 30 to 60 seconds in most cases.

Irrespective of the cause of cardiac arrest, if irreversible cerebral damage or death is to be prevented, CPR must be started immediately. For if, in primary cardiac arrest, the onset of reoxygenation by CPR is delayed beyond about 5 minutes, the chances of recovery without brain damage are small, unless special brain resuscitation measures are employed (Chapter III). This time interval is slightly longer in hypothermic patients, those who have taken certain drugs and in young children.

Recognition of Cardiac Arrest (Fig. 25)

Cardiac arrest is *defined* as «the clinical picture of sudden cessation of circulation in a patient who was not expected to die at that time». Cessation of circulation is diagnosed when all the following conditions are present: *unconsciousness; apnea or gasps; deathlike appearance* (cyanosis or pallor); and *absence of pulse in large arteries* (e.g., carotid or femoral). Pulselessness of the carotid artery is the most important of these signs (Fig. 25) and is to be favored over absence of heart sounds, an unreliable sign. Notably, peripheral pulses may be absent in spite of the presence of the carotid pulse.

Palpation of the femoral artery, however, is an acceptable means of checking for the presence or absence of pulses, although it is chiefly applicable to hospitalized patients.

In *infants* and small *children*, the carotid pulse may also be felt, but this easily compresses the airway or causes laryngospasm. Thus, determine pulselessness by feeling the brachial or femoral artery, the abdominal aorta, or the ventricular beat over the precordium.

Although dilated pupils are sometimes listed as an additional sign, one should not wait for pupils to dilate, since this may take more than one minute after cessation of circulation to occur. In some patients in cardiac arrest the pupils never dilate at all. Drugs may alter pupil size and reaction. Relative changes in pupil size can, however, be valuable in following the effectiveness of artificial circulation and the course of post-resuscitation recovery.

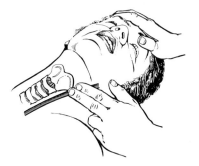

Figure 25: Feeling for the carotid pulse to determine pulselessness
Maintain backward tilt of the head with one hand, while feeling for the patient's carotid pulse with your other hand. Check the side of the patient's neck closest to you; do not reach over his neck, as this maneuver is awkward and may, as well, occlude the patient's airway. Feel for the pulse by placing your index and middle fingers gently on the patient's larynx (Adam's apple); then slide the fingers off to the side and press gently backward on his neck. Palpate with the flat portion of your fingers, rather than with the tips. If you do this correctly, the carotid artery should lie beneath your fingers. When feeling the artery, take care not to occlude it. Palpate long enough (at least 10 seconds) to ensure that you do not miss a slow heart rate. Practice on normal patients.

Closed Chest Cardiopulmonary Resuscitation (Fig. 26, 27)
The rediscovery of *external cardiac compressions* (Kouwenhoven, Jude) and its combination with airway control and artificial ventilation have made it possible for any trained person to initiate attempts at reversal of clinical death, even outside the hospital.

The heart occupies most of the space between the sternum and the spine in the lower chest (Fig. 26). Artificial circulation is most readily produced by chest compressions, which may squeeze the heart between the sternum and the spine. Blood is thereby forced out of the heart, lungs and great vessels, producing some systemic and pulmonary circulation. When sternal pressure is released, the elasticity of the chest wall causes the thorax to expand and the chest, including the heart, refills with blood. Meanwhile the blood is oxygenated in the lungs.

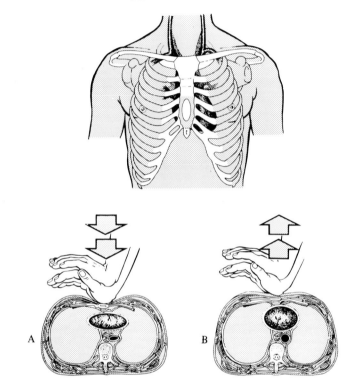

Figure 26: External cardiac compressions
Top: *The correct place for application of the hands, i.e., the lower half of the sternum.*
Bottom: *(a) Compression of chest between sternum and spine with heel of hand applied to the sternum. Second hand applied on top of the first hand. (b) Release of pressure to let chest fill. Compress and release for 50 per cent of each cycle. Maintain contact between hand and sternum.*

The *mechanism* by which external cardiac compressions move blood is under re-investigation. It has been known for a long time that forceful IPPV without sternal compressions can move a trickle of blood flow. Functional valving of large veins at the thoracic inlet (Weisfeldt) and diaphragm (Lesser) has been demonstrated. External cardiac compressions seem to move blood by variable combinations of 2 mechanisms: (1) direct *compression of the heart* (particularly when the heart is large and the chest is compliant; and (2) *overall intrathoracic pressure fluctuations* (chest pump), which can be augmented by IPPV simultaneously with chest compressions (Wilder, Harris, Weisfeldt).

Sternal compressions can produce systolic blood pressure peaks of 100 mmHg and more, but the diastolic pressure is usually not more than 10 mmHg and the systolic central venous pressure (and intracranial pressure) is increased almost as much as arterial pressure, leaving only a minimal perfusion pressure. (This is not the case in open chest cardiac compressions, during which venous pressure is not significantly increased) (DelGuercio, Bircher). External cardiac compressions result in a cardiac output and carotid artery blood flow of usually less than 30 per cent of normal flow, sometimes less than 10 per cent (Redding, DelGuercio, McKenzie, Harris, Bircher). This would not be enough to maintain or restore consciousness and can be borderline for maintaining

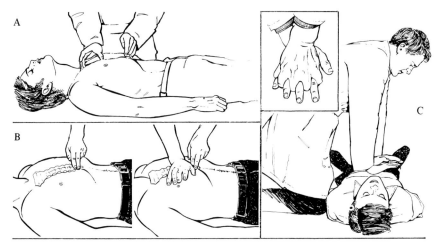

Figure 27: Technique of external cardiac compressions
(A) Identification of correct point for external cardiac compressions, by feeling for suprasternal notch and base of xiphoid, measuring one-half of this distance and compressing the lower half of the sternum.
(B) Alternative method for identifying the pressure point, i.e., feeling for the base of the xiphoid, measuring two fingers cephaled (left), and applying heel of hand over lower half of sternum (right).
(C) Body and hand position for external cardiac compressions. Compress straight downward, using part of body weight. Keep arms straight and hands off ribs. Inset: alternative method for performing external cardiac compressions with heel of lower hand, by locking fingers of both hands.

viability of cerebral neurons during prolonged CPR (Alifimoff).

For artificial circulation, *pressure* should be *applied* at exactly the lower half of the sternum in order to be effective and to avoid injury. The layman can be taught to recognize the sternum by feeling the abdomen, which is soft, and the sternum, which is hard.

The pressure point is identified by feeling for the xiphoid process (lower end of the sternum) and suprasternal notch (upper end of the sternum), and dividing in half the distance between them (Fig. 27 A).

Another method is feeling for the xiphoid process, and placing two fingers just above the base of the xiphoid process, and the heel of the other hand adjacent to the two fingers; this identifies the lower half of the sternum (Fig. 27 B).

The *technique* for artificial circulation is as follows (Fig. 27):
1 Position yourself to either side of the patient.
2 Locate the xiphoid-sternal junction.
3 Place the heel of one hand over the pressure point at the lower half of the sternum and place the heel of the other hand on top of the first hand.
4 Push the sternum downward toward the spine about 1 ½ to 2 inches (4 to 5 cm) in adults. The force required varies and should not be more than necessary for sternal displacement.
5 Hold the sternum down for about one-half second (50 per cent of the cycle). Then release rapidly and wait for another one-half second (other 50 per cent of the cycle) to let the chest fill with blood.
6 Reapply pressure every second or at a slightly faster rate. The presently recommended rate is 60 per minute for 2 operators (with ventilation interposed after every fifth compression) and 80 per minute for 1 operator (alternating 15 compressions with 2 quick lung inflations).

Compress the sternum forcefully enough to produce a good artificial carotid or femoral pulse. Bear in mind, however, that the pulse volume you feel does not necessarily reflect the degree of blood flow. Ask another member of the team to monitor the pulse produced by your compressions, witch should be regular, smooth, and uninterruped. Your arms should be vertical with elbows locked.

In adults, apply compression using your entire body weight with arms straight rather than arm muscles alone, to avoid fatigue. Do not lift your hands from the sternum between compressions, but do release pressure completely. Compress with the heels of your hands, keeping your fingers raised to avoid producing rib fracture by pressing against the lateral aspects of the thorax. Pressing below the xiphoid may cause regurgitation or rupture of the liver, and pressing too high may fracture the sternum.

The patient must be in the horizontal position to permit venous return, which may be promoted by raising the legs. The patient must also be on a firm surface (ground, floor, hard litter, spine board or — in the hospital — a cardiac arrest bed board). Cardiac compressions should not be delayed when such hard support is not immediately available. If the patient is in bed, do not waste time moving him to the floor, but slip a bed board or tray betwen his thorax and the mattress. Never interrupt compressions except for a few seconds, since even when optimally performed, they produce only borderline circulation.

In *small children,* compress the sternum with one hand only; in *infants* with the tips of two fingers.

In small infants, the rescuer may encircle the infant's chest with both hands and compress the midsternum with both thumbs.

The heart in infants and small children lies higher in the chest, and the danger of injuring the liver is greater; apply cardiac compressions over the midportion of the sternum. Press down only about one half inch (1 to 2 cm) in infants, and 1 to 1½ inches (2½ to 4 cm) in small children. In children and infants, compression rates of 100 to 120 per minute are recommended at present. Since backward tilt of the infant's head lifts his back, the back should be supported by one of the rescuer's hands, a folded blanket or other support. Most infants have an open airway with the head in the midposition.

Combinations of Ventilation and Sternal Compressions (Fig. 28, 29)
Sternal (chest) compressions alone can not provide ventilation of the lungs and therefore must be combined with IPPV.

The recommended *sequence* of CPR steps is thus as follows:

(A) If the patient is unconscious — tilt his head backward.

(B) If he is not breathing — ventilate his lungs rapidly three to five times; then quickly feel for his carotid pulse.

(C) If his pulse is present — continue ventilation at a rate of 12 per minute (one every five seconds); if his pulse is absent — start sternal (chest) compressions with recommended technique:

One-operator CPR (Fig. 28)
It is most important to teach this technique to all personnel, including the lay public, because rarely will there be more than one skilled bystander present at the scene at first.

Kneel at the patient's side (stand if he is on a litter, table, or bed).

Alternate two quick lung inflations with 15 sternal compressions. To obtain at least 60 sternal compressions per minute, perform each series of 15 compressions at a rate of about 80 compressions per minute. Deliver the two deep lung inflations (each 0.8 liter or more) — in rapid succession during five seconds, without allowing full exhalation to occur between breaths.

Maintain the patient's head tilted backward while ventilating and, if possible, raise his shoulders with a rolled blanket or hard object (e.g., special molded external cardiac compression board) to aid in maintaining the backward tilt.

Alternate rapidly between ventilation and sternal compressions. When ventilating by mouth-to-mask or bag-mask, strapping the mask to the patient's face loosely avoids delay due to frequent reapplications of the mask. Improvise your position trying to ventilate from your location at the side of the patient's head.

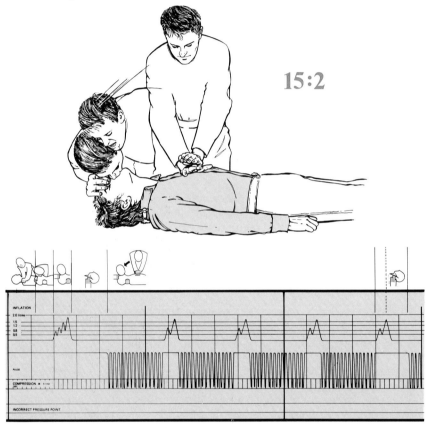

Figure 28: Combination *of artificial ventilation and artificial circulation for* **single operator** *without equipment using external CPR.*
Performance (top) and recording manikin print-out (bottom).

Technique:
If the victim is unconscious, tilt his head back. If he is not breathing spontaneously, give 3 to 5 quick lung inflations. Feel for a pulse for 5 to 10

seconds. If absent, give 15 chest compressions, then two quick lung inflations, and continue to alternate 15 compressions and two inflations. Perform external chest compressions at a rate of about 80 per minute (slightly faster than one per second) in order to produce at least 60 heart compressions per minute. Compress the sternum for 50 % of each cycle and release it for the other 50 %. Check for return of spontaneous pulse every 1—2 minutes.

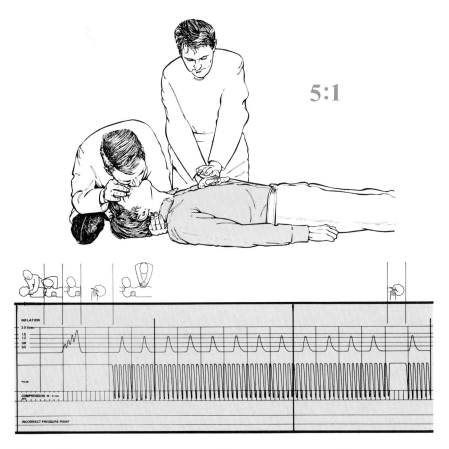

Figure 29: *External CPR sequence for **two operators** without equipment. Performance (top) and recording manikin print-out (bottom).*
(Two operators on opposite sides of patient).

Two operator CPR (Fig. 29)
This technique consists of continued uninterrupted chest compressions at a rate of one per second, i.e., 60 compressions per minute, with one lung inflation interposed after every fifth sternal compression.

Lung inflations should be interposed during the upstroke of each fifth chest compression. Interposing ventilations that quickly, in the patient without a tracheal tube requires much practice; therefore, this author favors use of the 2:15 ratio even when there are two operators, if the patient's trachea is not intubated.

One chest compression per second mitigates operator fatigue and allows inflations to be interposed without pauses. The two operators should position themselves on opposite sides of the patient, which permits easy changing of positions without interruption of the rhythm.

It should be stressed that there is nothing sacrosanct about these recommended rates and ratios of ventilation and sternal compressions. They are a compromise based on experimental data (Harris) and practical feasibility (Jude).

Technique:
Position yourselves on opposite sides of patient for easy switching of roles.

The first (ventilating) operator, tilt patient's head backward. Give 3 to 5 lung inflations. Feel for the pulse.

If pulse absent, second operator, start external chest compressions.

First operator, interpose one quick lung inflation after every fifth sternal compression, without interrupting compressions, at the rate of about one per second (60 per minute).

(In Fig. 29, for purposes of clear illustration, both rescuers are shown on the same side of the patient).

After endotracheal intubation, lung inflations may be uncoordinated with sternal compressions. Inflations can be interposed or simultaneous, but some interposed ventilations are required for lung expansion. Inflations simultaneous with chest compressions augment carotid flow (Wilder, Harris, Weisfeldt, Chandra). Because ventilations performed simultaneously with compressions require high airway pressures, they can be safely performed only via endotracheal tube.*

Augmentation of blood flow during external CPR is also possible by restraining the abdomen, by hand (Redding, Harris) or by pressure suit (military anti-shock trousers, MAST) (Bircher). These measures however can damage the liver and other abdominal organs and require high lung inflation pressures which require a tracheal tube (Bircher).* A safer method of augmentation of blood flow is an intravenous fluid load. Autotransfusion by the leg portion of the MAST is safe.

The new technique of high frequency positive pressure oxygen jet ventilation (Klain) makes synchronizing unnecessary, provides blood gas values comparable to IPPV, but does not augment blood flow.

For cough (self-induced) CPR, see Chapter IV.

*«New» CPR (Weisfeldt, Chandra, Rudikoff) is IPPVs simultaneously with each chest compression at 40 per minute (compression/relaxation time ratio 60/40%), plus abdominal restraint. «New» CPR augments *common* carotid artery blood flow as compared to standard CPR (Chandra), but increases intracranial pressure, which might worsen cerebral perfusion (Bircher). «New» CPR requires a tracheal tube (high airway pressure) and apparatus, and thus is *not* for basic life support. Pneumatic «new» CPR potentials for advanced life support or assistance of weak spontaneous circulation are being investigated.

Transition from One to Two Operators. The first operator had performed steps A and B, determined pulselessness, and initiated one-operator CPR with the ratio of 15 compressions followed by 2 inflations. If the second operator arrived after the first had initiated external cardiac compressions, he should identify himself, feel the carotid pulse generated by sternal compressions, and call out «stop compressions» to ascertain pulselessness for 5 seconds. If no pulse is found, the first operator continues external cardiac compressions and the second operator interposes ventilations after every fifth compression.

Switching between two operators. The two operators are on opposite sides of the patient, operator (1) ventilating, and (2) performing sternal compressions. When operator (2) gets tired, he replaces his normal cadence of «1-1000, 2-1000, 3-1000, etc» with «switch-on-three-next- time.» Immediately after «time», operator (2) gives the first 3 compressions of that cycle. The fourth and fifth compressions are taken over by operator (1). Operator (2) moves to the head and interposes ventilations 1:5. He should monitor his partner's sternal compressions by palpating the carotid artery. Alternatively, the deliberate five second pause in compressions for the purpose of evaluating the pulse may be used to effect a switch.

Monitoring the effectiveness of CPR. The ventilating operator should do this by (a) intermittently palpating the carotid pulse; and (b) by checking whether a spontaneous pulse has returned, at first after one minute of CPR and every few minutes thereafter, during brief interruptions of external cardiac compressions.

The pupils should also be examined periodically, as constriction and reaction to light indicate cerebral recovery, whereas fixed dilated pupils are an ominous sign as to the brain's status and the efficacy of CPR.

Continue CPR until a spontaneous pulse is restarted; with artificial ventilation continued until spontaneous breathing returns. Maintain oxygen therapy until the patient regains consciousness. While in ventricular fibrillation, a spontaneous pulse is not expected to return. In asphyxial cardiac arrest a spontaneous pulse usually returns rapidly without defibrillation after a few minutes of effective CPR.

External cardiac compression is an effective method of *mechanical pacing,* making the well oxygenated heart contract spontaneously in patients with heart block with severe bradycardia or asystole. However, since external cardiac compressions are painful, the conscious person with severe bradycardia is better treated with repetitive chest thumping (see «witnessed arrest») while waiting for the appropriate drugs and pacemaker insertion.

CPR Outside the Hospital. Ventilation and cardiac compressions should be well established by the manual technique before the victim is moved with manual or mechanical CPR. It is desirable that spontaneous circulation be restored at the scene, before moving the patient, but this depends on the availability of defibrillator, drugs, other equipment and personnel trained in advanced life support. If the patient must be moved for restoration of spontaneous circulation, a spontaneous pulse does not return with CPR, and drugs and defibrillator are not available, CPR must be continued without interruption during transport. This may prove difficult.

When moving the patient with manual CPR, the ventilating operator works from the head end of the stretcher, while the operator compressing the chest works from the side, and three or more bystanders carry the stretcher. The most experienced person present should act as team leader and coach the others.

When moving the patient over narrow stairways and other difficult routes, manual CPR will have to be improvised, but should not be interrupted for more than about 15 seconds at a time. A wooden backboard recommended for cases of suspected spine injury is also useful for transport of patients with CPR, provided the patient is strapped securely to the board.

In the ambulance, for one operator CPR, the operator kneels on a pillow near the side of the patient's head and chest, keeping the head tilted backward with a roll under the shoulder or use of a special backboard, which keeps the head tilted backward. A pharyngeal tube may be inserted and a transparent mask strapped loosely to the patient's face to avoid delays from frequent reapplications of the mask. The 2:15 ratio is used by the single operator, remaining at the side also for ventilation.

For the operator performing CPR in the ambulance, the astride position offers advantages over the conventional position (Fryer). The single operator facing cephaled (toward the patient's face) sits on a bench placed over the patient's hips and fastened to the stretcher. For ventilation, the operator pushes the chin upward (backward) to maintain head tilt when giving lung inflations via mask from a hand-triggered oxygen-powered ventilator or an improvised mouth-tube-valve-mask assembly.

Artificial circulation with the patient in the *upright position* (e.g., sitting, standing, hanging) is ineffective as the chest does not fill. Electric linemen who suffer cardiac arrest on the *poletop* should be lowered as quickly as possible for effective CPR on the ground, with some improvised CPR carried out during rescue.

External CPR machines (chest thumpers). CPR machines with mechanical ventilators attached are of value during difficult transport situations inside and outside hospitals. These machines provide more consistent CPR than can the manual technique, and about the same amount of blood flow. They can not «feel» like the operator's hand can and, therefore, if not ideally adjusted and constantly monitored may cause internal injuries. When CPR machines are used, manual CPR must be started first. «Thumpers» should be used only by personnel expertly trained in both manual and mechanical CPR, and fully drilled in the change to the mechanical device. Read the manufacturer's instructions carefully (Nobel).

These «chest thumpers» should provide an adjustable stroke of 1½ to 2 inches, be applied rapidly without interruption of manual CPR for more than 5 seconds at a time, support backward tilt of the head, and minimize the danger of accidental malpositioning of the plunger during use. When a mechanical device for ventilation is incorporated, it should be a volume- or time-cycled, not a pressure-cycled, ventilator. These devices are best employed with a cuffed endotracheal tube, since their ventilators do not adapt to the changing leaks and resistances usually encountered with ventilation by mask. Presently available «chest thumpers» are not suitable for infants and children. A rescuer must remain at the patient's head all the time to monitor plunger action and ventilation and to check the pulse and pupils.

The C-A-B Sequence Controversy. Some CPR educators in Europe recommend teaching 2 sequences: (1) Steps A-B-C, as described in this manual, for secondary arrest (e.g., asphyxia); and (2) Steps C-A-B for primary arrest (e.g., sudden cardiac death). The latter recommendation is based on the fact that in sudden cardiac arrest the arterial blood remains oxygenated for many minutes; it therefore could, according to this line of reasoning, be circulated with external cardiac compressions for the first 30 to 60 seconds, without delaying blood flow by Steps A and B. This proposal warrants further investigation. Deoxygenation during Step C is rapid.

In the meantime, a majority of existing guidelines continue to recommend the simple ABC sequence for both primary and secondary arrest, to avoid confusion. The difference between the two techniques may be more apparent than real, for in sudden cardiac arrest, the patient continues gasping for $\frac{1}{2}$ to 1 minute. This is a sign of brain stem perfusion and in itself might promote some blood flow. In such cases the need for Step A and B is obviated and the rescuer may proceed immediately to feeling the pulse and (if the pulse is absent) start external cardiac compressions. After 15 sternal compressions, the operator should ventilate 2 times and continue CPR.

Comment: When after initiation of closed-chest-CPR you cannot restore spontaneous circulation within a few minutes, try to augment cerebral and coronary bloodflow with IV fluids and epinephrine, simultaneous lung inflations and/or restraining the abdomen. If you are a physician trained in the method, do not hesitate to switch to *open-chest-CPR,* which is physiologically superior to any closed-chest method (see Chapter IV). CPR via thoracotomy is possible only in the hospital.

Control of Hemorrhage (Fig. 30, 31)
Circulation support in the bleeding patient with spontaneous pulse must start with controlling the hemorrhage.

Life-supporting first aid must be mastered by lay persons as well as health professionals. It includes head-tilt, jaw thrust, mouth-to-mouth ventilation, rescue pull, positioning for shock and coma, and measures to control external hemorrhage without surgical techniques, namely, by elevation, manual pressure and pressure bandage (Fig. 30).

Emergency care by *ambulance personnel* includes use of the tourniquet and control of internal hemorrhage below the diaphragm with use of the pressure suit, i.e., the «Medical (Military) Anti-Shock Trousers» (MAST) (Fig. 31) (Crile, Kaplan). These measures may also occasionally be indicated in intrahospital emergencies.

Emergency care by *physicians* of traumatized patients, goes beyond the scope of this manual. It includes clamping of bleeding arteries; pericardial drainage for cardiac tamponade; pleural drainage for pneumothorax and hemothorax; and resuscitative surgical operations for control of internal bleeding via thoracotomy, laparotomy or craniotomy. Fractures should be immobilized and soft tissue injuries protected against contamination; their definitive care however must not have priority over control of airway, breathing and bleeding, which must come first.

External hemorrhage must be controlled immediately since loss of one liter of blood or more in an adult (much less in children) can be lifethreatening.

If the patient is bleeding externally, elevate the bleeding site if possible (Fig. 30A) and apply manual pressure either directly or after covering the wound with sterile gauze to prevent infection (Fig. 30B)

Bleeding from veins and capillaries as well as most pulsating bleeding from arteries can be controlled by sealing with pressure the torn vessels against solid tissue underneath. Compressing arterial pressure points proximal to extremity wounds is less reliable and more difficult to learn.

If a pressure bandage is available (Fig. 30 C, D, E) and you cannot keep holding the wound until hospital admission, replace manual pressure with pressure by bandage. The pressure bandage shown in Fig. 30 consists of a sterile dressing pad, an elastic bandage strip to provide pressure and a semirigid styrene block to be placed directly over the bleeding site, with bandage strip and pad underneath. When the elastic bandage is wrapped over the styrene block, pressure is exerted against the wound, torn blood vessels are sealed and the bleeding stops (Laerdal).

To apply the pressure bandage, open the package, hold the bandage with both hands, place the dressing on the wound with the styrene block directly over the bleeding (Fig. 30 C).

Wrap the bandage over the styrene block several times. Do not tighten the bandage more than is necessary to stop the bleeding (Fig. 30 D).

Apply the final wrap loosely, press the end gently over the underlying wrap. The bandage is self-adhesive (Fig. 30 E).

If medical assistance is not immediately available, the pressure bandage should be loosened somewhat after about 30 minutes.

If you are the victim and alone, you can apply the pressure bandage on yourself.

Tourniquets should be used only as a last resort and only in cases of extremely traumatized extremities in which major vessels have been injured. Even in traumatic amputations, severed vessels usually retract and do not bleed. When the tourniquet is in place for extended periods, nerves, blood vessels and the entire extremity may be permanently damaged. When applied too loosely, the tourniquet can increase bleeding.

If you decide on using a tourniquet, use a cravat or folded handkerchief, not a rope or wire. Apply a pad over the artery to be compressed (pressure point). Wrap the tourniquet twice around the extremity and tie a half knot. Place a stick, pencil or similar object on top of the half knot and tie the ends of the tourniquet in a square knot above the stick. Twist the stick to tighten the tourniquet until the bleeding stops. Secure it in that position. Write on the patient's forehead «T» and the time the tourniquet was applied.

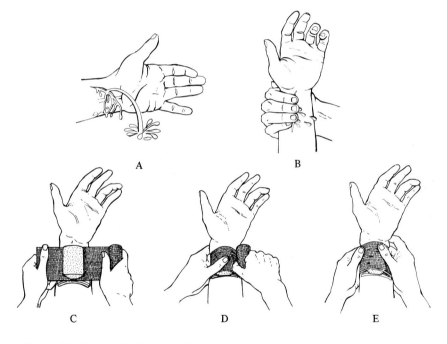

Figure 30: Control of external hemorrhage
(A) *Elevation of bleeding site.*
(B) *Direct manual pressure.*
(C) (D) (E) *Use of special pressure bandage (Laerdal).*
(C) *Application of dressing attached to elastic bandage and styrene block applied directly over bleeding site.*
(D) *Tightening of bandage over styrene block.*
(E) *Final wrap and fastening of bandage.*

Suspected internal hemorrhage below the chest can be treated nonsurgically in the prehospital setting with the *Medical Anti-Shock Trousers (MAST)* (Fig. 31) The MAST are a pressure suit which surrounds legs and abdomen. This pressure suit controls hemorrhage and provides autotransfusion in hypovolemic shock. It also effectively splints fractures of the pelvis and the lower extremities. Recommended inflation to about 100 mmHg intrasuit pressure can promptly reverse hypotension, presumably by mobilizing blood volume, compressing bleeding vessels, containing hematomas and perhaps even compressing the abdominal aorta.

Figure 31: *Application of the Military Anti-Shock Trousers (MAST). (from Armstrong Industries, Northbrook, Ill.; and Caroline N., Emergency Care in the Streets, Boston, Little-Brown publ., 1979).*

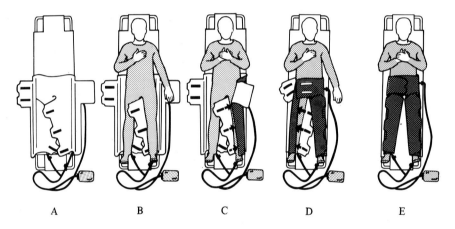

A	B	C	D	E

A. Unfold the MAST and lay flat (if stretcher is to be used lay MAST on it). Attach foot pump and open stopcock valves.
B. Put the patient on the MAST face up (supine), so that the top of the garment will be just below the lowest rib.
C. The left leg of garment is wrapped around the patient's left leg and secured with velcro strips.
D. The right leg of garment is wrapped around the patient's right leg and secured with velcro strips.
E. The material corresponding to the abdominal area is then put into place and secured with velcro strips.
   Using the foot pump, inflate the trousers until air exhausts through the relief valves and/or the patient's vital signs become stable.
   Close the stopcock valves.

During closed-chest *CPR*, the MAST can augment blood flow to the head. Use of leg garments is safe and sound (Caroline). Abdominal binding, however, can result in liver rupture between MAST and intrathoracic pressure (Bircher). Abdominal binding restrains the diaphragm; the patient should be given oxygen and, during CPR, may require intratracheal IPPV, because of a need for high inflation pressures. The MAST can cause renal ischemia (if in place longer than one hour) and pulmonary congestion, and can augment acidemia after its release.

abdominal section, then one leg section, and finally the other leg section, with 5 to 10 minute periods of titrated IV fluid administration in between. The MAST should not be removed until fluid resuscitation has started and the team is ready for resuscitative laparotomy, blood pressure support with vasopressor, and sodium bicarbonate to combat washout acidosis. If used for CPR, spontaneous cardiac action should be restarted prior to MAST release. In cases of suspected exsanguinating intra-abdominal arterial hemorrhage, as from ruptured aortic aneurysm, pressure with the fist on the upper abdominal aorta may be life saving, when MAST are not available. Some have applied effectively MAST in such cases and left them inflated until the thoracic descending aorta was clamped via thoracotomy (Stewart).

The MAST is relatively contraindicated in cases of head injury, suspected bleeding into the chest, or heart failure with pulmonary edema.

Extrication and Positioning for Shock (Fig. 32)

Circulation support in traumatic-hemorrhagic shock includes extrication of the patient from a wreck without adding injury, and positioning for shock. These measures must be preceded by ascertaining or controlling a patent airway and adequate breathing, and controlling external hemorrhage.

A seriously injured person should not be moved unless it is essential for lifesaving first aid, to avoid deterioration of injuries, or to protect him against further accidents.

When applying the *rescue pull,* move the injured limbs as little as possible; and immobilize the patient's head-neck-chest in the aligned position (Fig. 32 A) by yourself or by a helper.

When applying the rescue pull to a victim of a car accident, approach him from behind, place your arms under his armpits, grasp an unhurt arm, lift him gently, and drag him carefully along while you move backwards. While doing so, keep his head-neck-chest in the aligned position with his head in the mid-position, using your shoulder and chin or the aid of a bystander, who should hold his head with both hands. Avoid flexion, lateral rotation and maximal backward tilt of the head.

When pulled onto a flat surface, make him comfortable while waiting for the ambulance. Avoid unnecessary pain, protect him against cold and dampness.

Do not leave him alone. Reassure him. Check breathing frequently and stop bleeding. Dress major wounds.

«Rescue pull» (Fig. 32A) is extrication without equipment. However, ambulance personnel, whenever possible, should extricate with the help of a short backboard applied before moving the patient, and extricating him gently onto a long backboard, using established methods of prehospital emergency care (Caroline).

Shock is defined as «a reduction in overall tissue perfusion, resulting in vital organ systems malfunction». Trauma and other conditions which lead to external and/or internal blood volume loss produce the clinical picture of overall hypoperfusion — namely, cold moist skin, oliguria- anuria, tachycardia (may be absent in infancy, old age or during general anesthesia), faint peripheral pulses, arterial hypotension (blood pressure may be normal in fit persons unitl 20 to 30 % of blood volume has been lost because of compensatory vasoconstriction) and CNS excitation-depression.

If he is unconscious and breathing adequately, place him in the supported supine aligned position (Fig. 3A) or the stable side position (Fig. 3B) (pages 19, 20).

If he is conscious with signs of shock, keep him *horizontal* and supine (face-up) and elevate his legs (Fig. 32B). This may have a slight autotransfusion effect. Keep him warm, but avoid overheating. Light weight thermal blankets are useful. Head-down position is *not* recommended.

Do not give him anything to drink, as he may need anesthesia. Even when conscious, he may vomit and aspirate.

Prehospital and intrahospital advanced life support for patients with shock (fluid resuscitation and drugs) are covered in Chapter II.

Victims of trauma should be managed with life-supporting first aid and emergency care going hand-in-hand with *evaluation:*

Primary survey — Conscious? Airway? Breathing? Pulse?

Secondary survey — Pulse rate. Blood pressure. Respiration. Skin. Examine from head to toe, looking for wounds and fractures.

Primary survey by bystander, secondary survey by health care personnel.

In unconscious patient, with or without injury, look for *Medic Alert* bracelet or necklace. An underlying disease may call for modification of standard resuscitation procedures (e.g., allergies, diabetes, epilepsy).

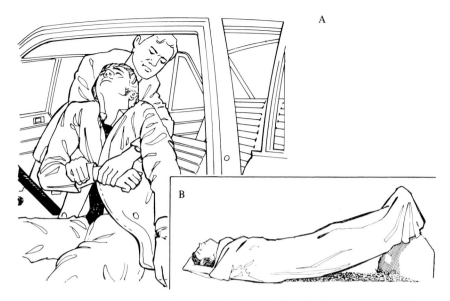

Figure 32: Rescue pull and positioning for shock. *(A) Rescue pull from behind, to remove victim from wreck, without aggravating his injuries, keeping head, neck and chest aligned (by a second rescuer, if available, holding the victim's head with both hands). (B) Positioning for shock — horizontal, with legs raised, head tilted backward and wrapped for warmth. (Do not overheat.)*

Comment: *A trickle of blood flow (near arrest) may be worse for cerebral recovery than no blood flow (Siesjo). About 10—20 % of normal cerebral blood flow, however, such as during CPR or in severe shock, while incapable of restoring consciousness, can maintain viability of neurons for some time (Steen). Such severe overall hypoperfusion, if prolonged, (30—60 minutes or more), can trigger irreversible multiple organ systems failure in spite of transiently «effective» resuscitation. Because of the importance of the **time factor** for ultimate intact survival, every effort must be made to immediately restart spontaneous circulation in cardiac arrest and, in the presence of spontaneous circulation, to combat any shock state without delay (Chapters II, III).*

ADVANCED LIFE SUPPORT
Restoration of Spontaneous Circulation

Chapter II

Spontaneous circulation should be restored as promptly as possible after initiation of basic life support, since external cardiac compressions produce only borderline blood flow, which may be inadequate to keep the brain and heart viable for longer than a few minutes of CPR. Restoration of spontaneous circulation usually requires intravenous (I.V.) administration of drugs and fluids *(Step D);* electrocardiographic diagnosis *(Step E);* and fibrillation treatment *(Step F)* — in varying sequences depending on circumstances. In ventricular fibrillation that occurs while a patient's EKG is being monitored, for example, electric countershock (Step F) should not be delayed by Steps D and E and precede steps A,B,C. Furthermore, none of the steps D, E and F will be required if a spontaneous pulse returns promptly following initiation of artificial ventilation and external cardiac compressions, as is often the case in pulselessness secondary to asphyxia. Needless to say, during attempts at restoring spontaneous circulation, oxygen transport by CPR (Steps A, B and C) must be maintained with as little interruption as possible.

DRUGS AND FLUIDS

Routes for Drugs and Fluids
Peripheral Intravenous Route (Fig. 33). A peripheral intravenous route for the administration of drugs and fluids should be established as quickly as possible after the initiation of CPR, but without interrupting CPR, in order to expand the circulating blood volume and provide a route for the administration of drugs. If an intravenous (I.V.) infusion is already running, drugs, fluids and glucose should be given via the existing route. If there is no infusion in place and if establishment of a percutaneous peripheral venous catheter is not immediately possible, the first I.V. injection of epinephrine (adrenalin) may be made via a small gauge needle into a peripheral vein (e.g., external jugular vein). Sodium bicarbonate, on the other hand, because it requires a large volume for injection, is better withheld until a reliable venous catheter has been inserted. Continuous infusion via metal needles is not recommended, as these are easily dislodged during CPR.

A member of the team not occupied with ventilation and cardiac compressions should start a peripheral venous infusion in an arm or leg vein, using the largest accessible vein for this purpose. An arm vein is first choice because infusions into leg veins are more likely to result in thromboses and delayed entry of drugs into the heart. For blood volume replacement, a catheter needle 16 gauge or larger is desirable; for drug administration any smaller size is acceptable. The technique of percutaneous peripheral venous cannulation is illustrated in Figure 33. A catheter- outside-needle or a catheter-inside-needle may be used, but the former causes less leakage of blood around the catheter and allows a larger diameter catheter to be inserted.

First choice is a vein you can feel. If a peripheral extremity vein is not palpable, the external jugular vein is good second choice; digital compression just above the clavicle distends the external jugular vein and renders it more easily cannulated.

Third choice is the femoral vein, although invisible; it is located in the inguinal region just medial to the femoral artery, whose pulsations are palpable during cardiac compressions. Finally, the last choice for the peripheral venous cannulation is a rapid venous cut-down.

Cut-down is usually more quickly and easily accomplished at the ankle (saphenous vein) than at the wrist or elbow, and can be executed rapidly by making a 2-3 cm transverse incision just anterior to the internal malleolus, then picking up the vein with a hemostat after blunt tissue dissection, inserting a large-bore needle or cannula into the vein, and clamping the vein distally. To save time, a large blunt metal cannula can be inserted via a small incision in the vein, and a hemostat can be placed over vein and cannula proximally. No other clamps or sutures are needed initially.

Attempts at cannulating subclavian or internal jugular veins for central venous catheterization are contraindicated during CPR steps ABC, because of the danger of inducing pneumothorax when these measures are attempted in the patient who is being bounced by cardiac compressions; furthermore, such measures may require interruption of CPR at a stage when priority must be given to ventilation, oxygenation and cardiac compressions. After spontaneous circulation has been restored, on the other hand, prolonged life-support measures (Phase III) do indicate the use of central venous and arterial catheters in most comatose patients. A pulmonary artery balloon catheter may be inserted in selected cases as well, after the patient is stabilized (see later).

Intrapulmonary Route. Intratracheal instillation of selected drugs is recommended in situations where an intravenous route is not readily available (Redding). Epinephrine, lidocaine (lignocaine, Xylocaine), atropine, and other drugs that do not cause tissue damage, can safely be given via the tracheal tube, using 1-2 times the intravenous dose, diluted in 10 ml of sterile water. Bicarbonate, however, must *not* be given

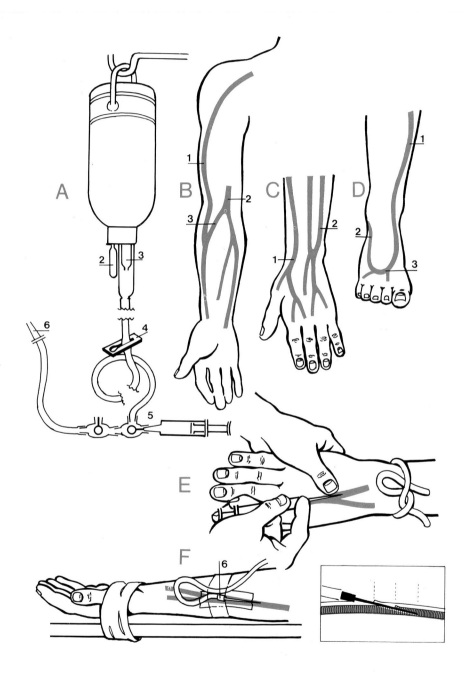

Figure 33: Technique of peripheral venous cannulation for intravenous infusion (from Dripps, R, et al., Introduction to Anesthesia, Saunders publ., 1975).

A. **Infusion apparatus:** *1, hook on pole of adjustable height; 2, air inlet; 3, drip bulb; 4, clamp for controlling flow of fluid; 5, adapter inserted into double three-way stopcocks with syringe for drugs or flushing (second stopcock for additional infusion); 6, adapter for insertion into catheter needle.*

B. **Veins of arm:** *1, cephalic; 2, basilic, 3, antecubital.*

C. **Veins of dorsum of hand:** *1, cephalic, 2, basilic.*

D. **Veins of dorsum of foot:** *1, great saphenous vein; 2, small saphenous vein; 3, dorsal venous arch.*

E. **Technique** *of venipuncture and insertion of catheter-outside-needle:*
  (1) apply venous tourniquet;
  (2) identify vein;
  (3) clean site with antiseptic solution;
  (4) pierce skin with needle; (see insert of F);
  (5) with second abrupt definitive but controlled motion pierce vein;
  (6) ascertain blood backflow;
  (7) advance catheter over needle, withdraw needle;
  (8) connect infusion to catheter; (see insert of F);
  (9) tape securely with transparent tape.
  *For catheter-inside-needle (not shown) use similar technique but **never** withdraw catheter from needle, as the sharp needle tip may shear off the end of the catheter, which can disappear into the venous system.*

F. **Fixation** *of intravenous catheter needle and tubing to arm, using transparent plastic tape at connector, same as 6 of picture A. Note loop of intravenous tubing and longitudinal tape to prevent inadvertent dislodgement.*

intratracheally, as it may damage the mucosa and alveoli. A drug instilled in this fashion is rapidly absorbed across the alveoli, particularly when the drug is injected into the tracheobronchial tree through a suction catheter inserted via the tracheal tube. The effect can be seen almost as rapidly as with I.V. administration.

Intracardiac Route. The blind intracardiac injection of drugs is *not* recommended during *closed* chest CPR, as it may produce pneumothorax, injury to a coronary artery and prolonged interruption of external cardiac compressions. Inadvertent injection into cardiac muscle rather than a cardiac chamber may, in addition, lead to intractable dysrhythmias. Intracardiac injection of epinephrine should be considered only in the rare instance that a vein is inaccessible, and the endotracheal route has not been established, and should be done via a long, thin (e.g., 22 gauge) needle through the fifth intercostal space parasternally into a heart chamber. The paraxyphoid approach (needle insertion to the left of the xyphoid process, and advancement cephalad, posteriorly, and laterally) is less likely to damage the anterior descending coronary artery. The position of the needle must be confirmed by free aspiration of blood, since intramyocardial injection can cause irreversible cardiac damage.

During *open* chest cardiac resuscitation, on the other hand, intracardiac injection is safe and effective if performed under direct vision. Epinephrine, antidysrhythmic agents and calcium have been effective when given into the left cardiac ventricle, in about one-half of the I.V. doses. Bicarbonate must not be given via the intracardiac route.

Intramuscular Route. One may also give the cardiac drugs lidocaine (300 mg) and atropine (2 mg) by intramuscular route for the *prevention* of dysrhythmias, under conditions where peripheral blood flow is adequate and I.V. administration is not possible. The intramuscular route, however, has no place in emergency resuscitation, because absorption of a given dose from the intramuscular site is unpredictable, and thus, the onset and duration of drug action cannot be reliably controlled.

Central Venous Route. As soon as possible after restoration of spontaneous circulation, a central venous catheter should be inserted to record central venous pressure (normal value 3-10 mm Hg), to offer an additional route for infusion, and to permit sampling of blood for various analyses.

The superior vena cava is the vessel of choice for central venous catheterization. A catheter in the superior vena cava is less dysrhythmogenic than one in the right atrium or pulmonary artery. Moreover, when mixed venous blood analysis is desired (for instance to follow oxygen values), superior vena cava blood is more representative of pulmonary artery blood, than samples from the inferior vena cava or the right atrium.

Many consider the *right internal jugular vein* the preferred approach to superior vena cava catheterization. The technique for cannulation through the right internal jugular vein includes turning the patient's head to the left side, palpating the carotid artery with one hand and inserting a catheter needle just lateral to the carotid artery, in a paramedian plane, 45 degrees caudad, piercing the skin at the superior tip of the triangle created by the two portions of the sternocleidomastoid muscle. As with any vascular cannulation, one can either insert a short large-bore metal needle and thread through it a smaller-bore catheter; or use a small-bore short catheter-outside-needle first, thread a guide wire through it, then remove the short needle and insert the long CVP catheter over the guide wire. The latter technique causes less leakage around the catheter. Strict asepsis is mandatory. In all central venous cannulations, one must guard against air embolism whenever the system is open to the atmosphere: the patient's head should be slightly lowered; the conscious patient should be asked to hold his breath, while the unconscious patient should receive positive pressure ventilation; and, during unavoidable periods of disconnection, the opening should be occluded by finger or stopcock.

Catheterization of the right internal jugular vein does not require X-ray control since the catheter reliably passes into the superior vena cava. However, when the superior vena cava is catheterized via an arm vein (basilic or cephalic vein) or the subclavian vein, the catheter sometimes passes into the opposite arm or the jugular vein; thus X-ray check of catheter position is desirable. However, central venous catheterization from the right arm (with the patient's head leaned to the right), is a fairly reliable second choice route. Catheterization through the subclavian vein, despite its popularity, remains a definite last choice, for its use is still associated with a high incidence of complications, such as pneumothorax and mediastinal infusion.

Pulmonary Artery Catheterization. A pulmonary artery catheter is rarely needed during Phase II of emergency resuscitation; however, it is a useful adjunct for selected cases during long-term life support. The value of pulmonary artery catheterization must in each case be weighed against associated potential complications, which include life-threatening dysrhythmias and distraction of team effort from more important and simpler life support measures. Insertion of a pulmonary artery balloon catheter (Swan-Ganz) is indicated to monitor pulmonary artery wedge pressure (a reflection of left atrial pressure) in left ventricular failure; to titrate major fluid therapy in patients with alveolar-capillary membrane leakage or renal failure; to determine whether increased pulmonary artery pressure is the result of increased pulmonary vascular resistance or of left ventricular failure; and to determine whether increased CVP is due to right or left heart failure. The pulmonary artery catheter also permits monitoring of mixed venous PO_2 (normal value 40-50 mm Hg) and oxygen content. A reduction of pulmonary artery PO_2, with arterial PO_2 unchanged, suggests a decrease in arterial oxygen transport (blood flow times oxygen content) below that required for the patient's oxygen consumption. Finally, a pulmonary artery catheter, used in concert with an arterial catheter, facilitates monitoring of cardiac output by the thermodilution technique. Pressure measurements, however, are the main indication for pulmonary artery catheterization. Normal pulmonary art. press. is $25/10$ mm Hg, mean 15 (range $14-17$) mm Hg. Normal mean pulmonary artery wedge pressure (during occlusion of the peripheral pulmonary artery, reflecting left atrial pressure) is 10 (6-12) mm Hg. Pulmonary artery wedge pressure should not be permitted to exceed plasma colloid osmotic (oncotic) pressure, which normally is 25 mm Hg, but can be significantly reduced in severe illness or injury. Monitoring of plasma colloid osmotic pressure (or at least albumin concentration) is desirable in long-term resuscitation.

Arterial Puncture and Catheterization (Fig. 34). Catheterization of a peripheral artery is indicated for patients requiring long-term life support measures and repeated blood gas determinations over an extended period. The placement of an arterial catheter is *not* part of the initial stages of resuscitation, but should be inserted only after restoration of spontaneous circulation, in a patient who does not show signs of regaining consciousness.

For initial blood gas determinations, arterial puncture is sufficient. Although arterial puncture is feasible during cardiac compressions (particularly using the femoral artery), it does not have high priority at this stage of resuscitation, and should not interfere with more fundamental therapeutic measures. As soon as possible after restoration of spontaneous circulation, however, an arterial blood sample of about 0,5 ml should be drawn for determination of PO_2, PCO_2, pH and hematocrit. Emergency hospitals receiving resuscitation cases should have STAT blood gas laboratory services available 24 hours a day.

Arterial puncture is best accomplished using a small, heparin-rinsed syringe with a 25 gauge needle. The radial artery is the site of choice for arterial sampling, since asepsis is more easily assured at that site than in the groin and subsequent bleeding may be more readily controlled. The patency of the ipsilateral ulnar artery should be confirmed before radial artery puncture (Allen's test). Blood samples should be drawn bubble-free into the prepared syringe. If any delay in processing the sample is anticipated, the syringe should be placed in ice.

When long-term *arterial catheterization* is indicated, we recommend the femoral artery (Fig. 34). Radial artery catheterization with a 20-22 gauge catheter-outside-neddle is safe, but only if the catheter is left in place for less than 1-2 days; thereafter the risk of thrombotic occlusion increases significantly. For femoral artery catheterization, the puncture site near the inguinal ligament lies between the femoral vein medially and the femoral nerve laterally.

Under sterile technique, the femoral artery is palpated, a 16 gauge needle is inserted and a 18 gauge catheter fed through the needle into the lower abdominal aorta and held firmly in place. The needle is withdrawn over the catheter. The alternative technique with guide wire may also be used. Connections to stopcocks for sampling-flushing and to the strain gauge must be nonslipping (locking) to prevent exsanguinating hemorrhage. A continuous flushing device is safer than intermittent flush. Patency can be maintained for weeks by keeping a dilute heparin solution in the catheter (10 mg or 1000 units of heparin in 500 ml isotonic saline).

Meticulous aseptic, bubble-free, clot-free technique is essential for all vascular cannulations.

The arterial route should *not* be used for the administration of drugs and fluids, because of the potential for inducing embolic-thrombotic complications.

For details of vascular catheterizations, see:

(a) Safar, P. et al.: Principles and Practice of Emergency Medicine. Chapters 9 and 10. Philadelphia, Saunders publ., 1978; 1984.

(b) Shoemaker, W.C. and Thompson, W.L. (editors): Critical Care, State of the Art, Society of Critical Care Medicine, 223 East Imperial Highway, Suite 140, California 92635, USA; 1980-81.

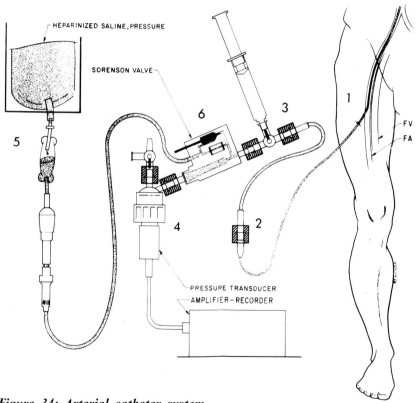

Figure 34: Arterial catheter system
Femoral artery catheter (1) connected via nonslipping adaptors (2) and three-way stopcock with sampling syringe (3) to pressure transducer (4). Interposed flushing system (5) with heparin (10 mg or 1000 units / 500 ml saline) under pressure and Sorenson valve (6), permitting slow, continuous flush plus intermittent manual flush.

Drugs

Drugs during Cardiac Compressions

Epinephrine (adrenalin) and sodium bicarbonate may help restore spontaneous circulation in cardiac arrest of more than about 1-2 minutes duration, irrespective of the electrocardiographic (EKG) pattern, i.e., ventricular fibrillation, ventricular tachycardia, electrical asystole, or electromechanical dissociation (mechanical asystole with bizarre EKG complexes). In cases of persistent or recurrent ventricular fibrillation or ventricular tachycardia without a pulse — in spite of effective CPR, correctly applied countershock, and normal blood gas and pH values — lidocaine (Xylocaine, lignocaine) and if ineffective, bretylium are also indicated during cardiac compressions. Other drugs described below are for the pre- or post-arrest period.

Witnessed, EKG Monitored Arrest — Ventricular Tachycardia or Fibrillation

1 If a defibrillator is immediately available, administer external electric countershock within 30 seconds of the patient's collapse. Do not delay countershock for administration of drugs or CPR-ABC.
2 If the first countershock fails to restore a spontaneous pulse immediately, start closed-chest CPR and repeat countershocks every 1-2 minutes.
3 Give epinephrine 0.5—1.0 mg I.V. (adult dose), followed by sodium bicarbonate 1 mEq/kg I.V. as soon as possible after the initiation of CPR-ABC. If countershock has failed, circulate the drugs by cardiac compressions for at least one minute before repeating countershock. Do not use bicarbonate if there has been prompt initiation of CPR and minimal tissue acidosis, as it may lead to alkalemia with intractable ventricular fibrillation.
4 If countershock fails to convert the rhythm or if a spontaneous pulse is achieved but then reverts rapidly to ventricular fibrillation or ventricular tachycardia, give lidocaine 100-200 mg by *slow* I.V. push, followed by an infusion of lidocaine 1-3 mg per minute (adult dose). Then repeat countershock.

Witnessed Arrest — Asystole or Electromechanical Dissociation (EKG)
Unwitnessed Arrest

1 Start CPR-ABC as soon as possible.
2 Give epinephrine 0.5—1.0 mg I.V. (adult dose). (Dilution is not necessary). Repeat this dose, or even a larger dose (1-2 mg) every 2-5 minutes. (If there is no intravenous route available, give the epinephrine via needle puncture of a peripheral vein, or via the endotracheal route, as described earlier).
3 When cardiac arrest has lasted 2 minutes or longer, or tissue hypoxia

has existed prior to arrest, give sodium bicarbonate, 1 mEq/kg I.V., slowly into a running infusion. In these circumstances, sodium bicarbonate combats the acidemia that would otherwise offset epinephrine's action.

4 One half of the above dose of bicarbonate may be repeated «blindly,» but not more than every 5-10 minutes of CPR, lest alkalemia and hyperosmolality develop. Once arterial pH values are available, bicarbonate administration should be guided by such measurements and accompanied by moderate hyperventilation.

The reason for recommending epinephrine first and bicarbonate second is based on the practical fact that the small volume of epinephrine is easily and rapidly administered into a peripheral vein. The longer time taken to infuse the larger volume of bicarbonate, which must be given slowly, should not be permitted to delay the early effect of epinephrine. In cases of cardiac arrest secondary to asphyxia or exsanguination, and in cases of asystole following electric defibrillation, restoration of spontaneous circulation is usually enhanced by administration of epinephrine I.V., and enhanced further when sodium bicarbonate is added (particularly·in arrest periods longer than about 2 minutes), but is not enhanced by sodium bicarbonate alone (Kirimli). Occasionally epinephrine given in asystole may provoke ventricular fibrillation; this calls for external electric countershock.

In cardiac arrest no drug is effective without IPPV and cardiac compressions; and in *monitored* arrest with ventricular fibrillation or ventricular tachycardia, immediate electric countershock has priority over drugs. In *unwitnessed* arrest and ventricular fibrillation diagnosed by EKG, early countershock usually results in asystole rather than sinus rhythm, because of severe acidosis.

Drugs for CPR need reinvestigation. At the present time their use is as much an art as a science. Drug administration must be on a skillfully titrated basis, in concert with CPR, countershocks and fluid administration — with a feeling of utmost urgency to minimize interruptions of artificial circulation and ventilation and to restore spontaneous circulation as early as possible.

Epinephrine (Adrenalin)

This historic cardiovascular stimulant (Crile) is still unsurpassed by other sympathomimetic amines for use during cardiac arrest and CPR, because of its combined strong alpha-receptor and beta-receptor stimulating effects. The alpha-receptor stimulating effect of epinephrine increases systemic peripheral vascular resistance (without constricting the coronary and cerebral vessels), raises systolic and diastolic pressures during cardiac compressions, and thereby improves myocardial and cerebral blood flow, which in turn facilitates the return of spontaneous cardiac contractions. The beta-receptor stimulating effect of epinephrine (increased contractile state of the heart) is probably less important during cardiac compressions, but may become advantageous once spontaneous cardiac contractions resume. The combined alpha and beta effects give a high initial cardiac output and arterial pressure at the beginning of spontaneous reperfusion, which benefits cerebral and other vital organ system blood flow.

In asystole, epinephrine helps restart spontaneous cardiac action, as it elevates perfusion and increases myocardial contractility. In pulselessness with bizarre EKG complexes (electromechanical dissociation), epinephrine often restores a spontaneous pulse. Although epinephrine can produce ventricular fibrillation, particularly in the non-beating unevenly anoxic (diseased) heart, it also renders the heart in ventricular fibrillation or ventricular tachycardia easier to defibrillate and subsequently start cardiac contractions. In the presence of ventricular fibrillation, epinephrine converts fine ventricular fibrillation into coarse (strong) ventricular fibrillation, which is again more suspectible to termination by electric countershock. Furthermore, epinephrine increases the likelihood that adequate spontaneous circulation will resume after successful countershock.

During CPR-ABC, epinephrine 0.5-1.0 mg (adult dose) should be given I.V. The first dose should be given without waiting for EKG diagnosis, and this dose should be repeated every 3-5 minutes, as the duration of action of epinephrine is short. If the I.V. route is impossible, the intratracheal route (see above) should be used (1-2 mg in 10 ml of water). Do not mix epin. and bicarbonate in same syringe.

After restoration of spontaneous circulation, a continuous I.V. infusion of epinephrine (1 mg in 250 ml) may be used to increase and sustain arterial pressure and cardiac output, starting with 0.5-1 micrograms per minute, and adjusted according to response. However, other sympathomimetic drugs are more commonly used after restoration of spontaneous circulation. To prevent recurrence of ventricular tachycardia or ventricular fibrillation during administration of a sympathomimetic amine, a simultanoeus infusion of lidocaine or bretylium has been suggested.

Other Sympathomimetic Amines (see below)
They do not seem to have significant advantages over epinephrine for use during CPR-ABC. Sympathomimetic amines with primarily alpha-receptor stimulating properties, such as norepinephrine (Levophed, noradrenalin) and metaraminol (Aramine), and drugs which are pure alpha-receptor stimulants such as phenylephrine (Neosynephrine) or methoxamine (Vasoxyl, Vasoxine), are also effective in raising diastolic arterial pressure during cardiac compressions and in facilitating restoration of spontaneous circulation in asystole (Redding, Pearson, Yakaites, Otto). They do not, however, provide an additional cardiac stimulating effect which may be desirable upon return of spontaneous

circulation. Also they have not yet received the extensive clinical attention that epinephrine has. Pure beta-receptor stimulating sympathomimetic amines, such as isoproterenol (Isuprel, isoprenaline), low-dose dopamine and dobutamine, as well as calcium, do not seem to aid in the restoration of spontaneous circulation; they lack the ability to increase arterial pressure during cardiac compressions.

Norepinephrine (Levophed, noradrenalin)
This naturally occurring catecholamine is primarily an alpha-receptor stimulant and the most potent vasopressor, secondary only to angiotensin II. It also exerts a slight beta-receptor activity. For use during CPR and cardiac compressions, prior to restoration of spontaneous circulation, norepinephrine may be given in the same doses as epinephrine and is effective in helping to restore spontaneous circulation (Smetana). Experience with norepinephrine in this setting is, however, limited.

Norepinephrine is less likely than epinephrine to produce recurrent tachydysrhythmias. Therefore some prefer it over epinephrine and dopamine for arterial pressure support *after* restoration of spontaneous circulation. When norepinephrine is given to the point of excessive vasoconstriction, renal and mesenteric blood flow are compromised and a severe metabolic acidosis may develop. The heart rate may slow due to a carotid baroreceptor reflex if hypertension occurs. When, however, in the presence of normovolemia, norepinephrine is cautiously infused merely to maintain normotension, clinical experience indicates that urine flow continues and no evidence of tissue ischemia is found. Control of arterial pressure and heart rate can be effectively accomplished by the combined administration of norepinephrine and isoproterenol (alpha + beta receptor stimulants).

Prolonged administration of norepinephrine in *hypovolemia* therefore is *contra-indicated*. However, in severe hemorrhage with profound hypotension, if there is delay in replacement of blood volume, particularly in elderly patients, coronary and cerebral perfusion can be protected, and cardiac arrest thereby prevented, by *brief* arterial pressure support with a vasopressor. Volume replacement must be started as soon as possible. In patients with ischemic heart disease, arterial pressure should not be raised above normal.

In the presence of spontaneous circulation with reduced peripheral resistance and hypotension, norepinephrine is given by titrated I.V. infusion, for example by adding 8 mg of norepinephrine to 500 ml of intravenous solution (yielding a concentration of 16 micrograms per ml), using a microdrip or infusion pump. One may start with 3 micrograms (0.2 ml)/minute per 70 kg. Because the effect of norepinephrine is potent, continuous arterial pressure monitoring is desirable. Infusion should be, if possible, via a central vein, since sloughing of superficial tissues may result from extravasation of norepinephrine around superficial venipunctures. If extravasation does occur, phentolamine should be infiltrated at the site.

Metaraminol (Aramine)

This drug has primarily alpha- and some beta-receptor stimulating action, but is less potent than epinephrine or norepinephrine. It exerts its effect by releasing catecholamine tissue stores, and thus is relatively ineffective in situations where such tissue stores are depleted, such as under the influence of reserpine, guanethidine, chronic heart failure or cardiac arrest. Metaraminol does not usually cause tachycardia and is useful as a mild vasopressor, even for prolonged administration. It is given by titrated I.V. infusion of a 0.4 mg/ml solution (100 mg in 250 ml). It can also be given by I.V. bolus of 1-5 mg.

Isoproterenol (Isuprel, Isoprenaline)

This is a sympathomimetic amine with pure beta-receptor stimulant action. Because of its lack of peripheral vasoconstricting action, it does not seem to enhance cerebral and coronary perfusion during cardiac compressions, and thus does not by itself lead to restoration of spontaneous circulation (Redding, Pearson, Yakaites). Indeed, it dilates peripheral vessels and thereby decreases perfusion pressure. While isoproterenol exerts a potent chronotropic and inotropic effect on the heart, resulting in increased cardiac output, at the same time it increases myocardial oxygen requirements. For these reasons, isoproterenol has no place during cardiac compressions, except perhaps in the case of asystole or severe atropine resistant bradycardia from heart block (Stokes-Adams syndrome), pending pacemaker insertion. Even in these cases, however, epinephrine is preferred for restarting the heart.

In myocardial infarction with spontaneous circulation and in cardiogenic shock, isoproterenol may increase myocardial oxygen requirements, leading to extension of the infarction; it is thus less beneficial for decreasing «after-load» than pure peripheral vasodilators such as nitroglycerin. Isoproterenol also may induce life-threatening tachydysrhythmias. If isoproterenol is administered, as for the treatment of heart block, it should be given by titrated I.V. infusion of 2-20 micrograms per minute, using a solution of 1 mg in 500 ml. The infusion is adjusted to keep the heart rate at about 60 per minute.

In status asthmaticus, where it is given for its beta effect on bronchi, an I.V. infusion of either isoproterenol of epinephrine may be «pushed» to the point of moderate tachycardia in an attempt to open the intrapulmonary airways. This treatment of asthmatic crisis, however, is a last resort, after measures with less risk to induce ventricular fibrillation have failed, i.e. IPPV with oxygen; metaproterenol (a beta-2 receptor stimulant); aminophylline I.V.; steroid I.V.; and arterial pH normalization.

Calcium

This physiologically important cation is essential for excitation-contraction coupling in muscle. Since calcium increases myocardial contractility it was tried in the early years of CPR instead of epinephrine, but proved to be less effective in the restoration of spontaneous circulation, since it does not cause peripheral vasoconstriction (Redding). Calcium is recommended for electromechanical dissociation, when epinephrine has failed to restart spontaneous cardiac action. Calcium, however, can cause coronary spasm and also increases myocardial irritability. Moreover, exessive doses may cause the heart to stop in contraction, particularly in the fully digitalized patient. The usefulness of calcium in resuscitation is doubtful (Dembo). It may be more appropriate than the sympathomimetic amines for use in cardiac depression from certain drugs such as barbiturates, but conclusive evidence is lacking. The preferred salt is calcium chloride 10 per cent, given in a dose of 5 ml/70 kg, and repeated if necessary at 10 minute intervals. Since 1 ml of the 10 per cent solution (100 mg of salt) contains 1.36 mEq of ionized calcium, the 5 ml dose contains 6.8 mEq. Other compounds used include calcium gluconate, given in a dose of 10 ml of a 10 per cent solution (4.8 mEq); and calcium gluceptate 5 ml of a 10 per cent solution (4.5 mEq). Calcium must not be given in the bicarbonate infusion, as the two react to form an insoluble precipitate of calcium carbonate.

Calcium Antagonists (e.g. Verapamil, Flunarazine).

These are being investigated for their promising coronary dilator, myocardial and cerebral protective and antifibrillation effects (Resnekov).

Dopamine.

This sympathomimetic amine is a biologic precursor of norepinephrine. It exerts dose-dependent cardiac inotropic action (beta- receptor stimulant) in low doses, and vasoconstrictor action (alpha-receptor stimulant) in high doses. Response differs between individuals and with dose and rate of administration (Goldberg). Its vasopressor potency is less than that of norepinephrine. Dopamine is more likely to dilate than constrict renal and mesenteric vessels, in doses which may not increase heart rate or blood pressure (1-2 micrograms/kg per minute). It is usually given by titrated I.V. infusion of a solution containing 200 mg of dopamine in 250 ml of 5 per cent dextrose in water (800 micrograms per ml). Slow infusion (2-10 micrograms/kg per minute) has primarily inotropic and renal vasodilating effects, but even at these low doses, dopamine may produce severe tachycardia. Rapid infusion or high concentrations (doses greater than 10 micrograms/kg per minute) exert an additional vasoconstrictor effect; and in doses above 20 micrograms/kg per minute even the renal and mesenteric vessels may be constricted.

The principal use of dopamine is in the support of perfusion pressure and cardiac output in cardiogenic or septic shock, using infusion rates of 2-5 micrograms/kg per minute. The infusion rate is increased until arterial pressure and urine flow respond. In CPR cases dopamine is useful for supporting arterial perfusion pressure after restoration of spontaneous circulation, once the more potent norepinephrine is no longer required. As when administering any vasopressor, normovolemia or slight blood volume expansion should be established. In cardiogenic shock oliguria may respond to furosemide better when arterial pressure is also supported by dopamine. Dopamine infusion should be discontinued gradually.

Dobutamine

This is a new synthetic catecholamine with beta-receptor stimulating action similar to that of isoproterenol (Tuttle). Its alpha(vasoconstrictor) effect even with large doses is minimal. It is not therefore surprising that it has been found to be inferior to epinephrine and high-dose dopamine for promoting restoration of spontaneous circulation during cardiac arrest (Otto). In high doses it can produce ventricular tachycardia. Dobutamine has been used by titrated I.V. infusion of 2.5-10 micrograms/kg per minute (maximum dose 20 micrograms/kg per minute) in refractory cardiogenic shock. It has also been used in conjunction with reduction of afterload by nitroprusside. Claims of advantages of dobutamine over isoproterenol or low-dose dopamine are not convincing, although less tachycardia may occur with dobutamine.

Sodium Bicarbonate

This is the second drug to be given during CPR (after epinephrine), in an initial dose of approximately 1 mEq/kg I.V. The purpose of administering sodium bicarbonate is to neutralize the fixed acids from ischemic tissue after circulatory arrest and during the borderline perfusion of CPR (Stewart). Severe acidemia should be reversed because it reduces the effect of epinephrine, and causes vasodilation, myocardial depression and capillary leakage. However, excessive sodium bicarbonate can cause metabolic alkalemia, impaired oxygen release from hemoglobin, ventricular tachycardia and fibrillation and sustained contraction (stone heart), and may also be injurious be producing hypernatremia with hyperosmolality (Mattar). During CPR less sodium bicarbonate is needed than previously assumed, whereas more is needed after restoration of spontaneous circulation when washout of acids increases. During CPR, acidemia can usually be corrected by moderate hyperventilation alone. Further hyperventilation is needed during sodium bicarbonate administration, since that drug forms CO_2. Without hyperventilation, sodium bicarbonate may paradoxically lower brain pH, even as it raises blood pH, because CO_2 passes through the blood-brain-barrier more readily than the charged bicarbonate or hydrogen ions (Bishop).

The recommended initial dose of sodium bicarbonate is 1 mEq/kg I.V. It should *not be given in the same infusion with epinephrine,* since it may inactivate the epinephrine in the solution. Bicarbonate is usually available in a solution of 1 mEq/ml in prefilled syringes, bottles or bags.

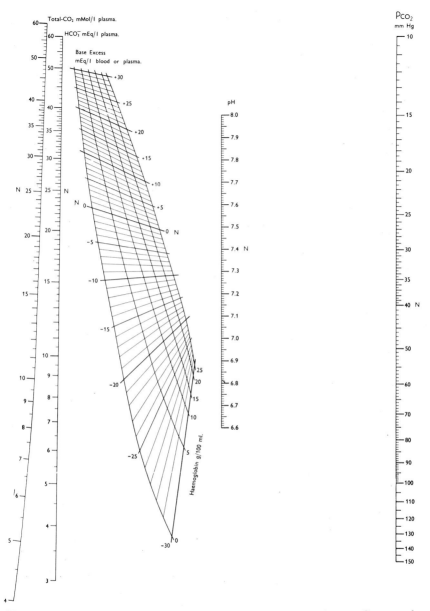

Figure 35: Blood acid-base alignment nomogram *according to Siggaard-Andersen. Measure blood PCO_2 and pH with appropriate electrodes. Connect values and read bicarbonate concentration in milliequivalents per liter (left). Determine hemoglobin and read base-excess where PCO_2-*

pH- bicarbonate line crosses the base-excess nomogram at the appropriate hemoglobin concentration. N: normal. This nomogram is designed for use with blood 38°C. (From Siggaard-Andersen: Scan. J. Clin. Lab. Invest., 15:211, 1963; also see Severinghaus, J.: Chapter 61 in Handbook of Physiology, Vol. II, Sec. 3, Respiration. American Physiology Society, 1965).

Additional blindly administered doses should not exceed 0.5 mEq/kg every 5 to 10 minutes of CPR. Ideally subsequent administration should be guided by arterial pH measurements, aiming for values near 7.4 (7.3-7.5).

Immediately after restoration of spontaneous circulation, the release of large amounts of carbonic acid and lactic acid from tissues calls for more hyperventilation and more bicarbonate, titrated according to arterial pH values (Figure 35). The optimal approach requires continuous adjustment of ventilation volumes to an arterial PCO_2 of 25-35 Hg; and use of sodium bicarbonate solely to correct base deficit.

Base deficit is calculated from arterial pH, PCO_2 and hemoglobin concentration, using the Siggaard-Andersen nomogram (Figure 35). *Calculation* of sodium bicarbonate dose requirements is performed as follows (Astrup):
1 Dose of bicarbonate = base deficit (mEq/liter) x (0.25) body weight (kg)

Example for 60 kg patient with base deficit of 10 mEq/liter — Bicarbonate dose required
= 10 mEq/liter x (0.25) (60) liters
= 10 mEq/liter x 15 liters
= 150 mEq
2 Give the first half of the above dose as a bolus I.V., and titrate the second half, only if needed, to reduce base deficit to 5 mEq/liter or less.

Tris buffer (THAM) has been used in lieu of and in the same dosage (in mEq) as sodium bicarbonate. THAM has the advantages of not being a CO_2 donor (and thus not requiring excessive hyperventilation) and entering the intracellular space more readily. However THAM has the disadvantages of not being available in a readily usable solution and causing apnea, hypoglycemia and venous irritation.

Lidocaine (Xylocaine, lignocaine)
This is the anti-dysrhythmic agent of choice for the treatment of premature ventricular contractions (PVCs) (ventricular ectopy, ventricular extrasystoles) — and for preventing progression to ventricular tachycardia or ventricular fibrillation.

Lidocaine was first introduced as a local anesthetic and later found to raise the ventricular fibrillation threshold (Carden). Lidocaine increases the electric stimulation threshold during diastole, and depresses cardiac irritability in cases of frequently recurring ventricular fibrillation. In equipotent antidysrhythmic doses, lidocaine produces less myocardial depression than other anti-dysrhythmic drugs.

Traditionally, lidocaine has been used where there are more than five PVCs per minute, short bursts of two or more PVCs in succession, PVCs of multiple configurations, or PVCs falling on the T wave, also called R-on-T phenomenon (Collinsworth). However, once myocardial ischemia is suspected, PVCs of any kind or frequency should be supressed with lidocaine. This drug is also the first choice during CPR when ventricular tachycardia or ventricular fibrillation is resistant to defibrillation.

Administration of Lidocaine

1 Give a loading dose of 1 mg/kg by slow IV bolus. (Some recommend 2-3 mg/kg.) This should be followed immediately by a continuous infusion of 1-4 mg/70 kg per minute, preferably via an infusion pump. Usually a solution of 1 mg/ml in 5% dextrose in water is used.

2 Additional boluses of 0.5-1.0 mg/kg may be given every five minutes, if necessary, to a total of 200-300 mg/70 kg.

The same mode of administration has been recommended as a primary prophylaxis against ventricular fibrillation, in cases of myocardial infarction. In intractable ventricular fibrillation, lidocaine should be used, but cannot alone — without electric countershock — convert ventricular fibrillation to a stable rhythm.

Side effects of lidocaine include myocardial depression, which is more likely to be apparent in the presence of cardiogenic shock; in such cases the normal bolus dose may be reduced by one half. Doses should also be reduced for patients with right heart failure, since clearance of lidocaine is delayed when there is passive congestion of the liver, and toxic levels of the drug may accumulate rapidly. Lidocaine may also cause central nervous system excitation (convulsions) or somnolence. Therefore, resuscitation equipment should be ready.

New *anti-dysrhythmic drugs* are under investigation (e.g., clofilium, amiodarone, verapamil). (Zipes, Resnekov).

Procaine (Novocain) *and Procainamide* (Pronestyl)

These drugs preceded lidocaine historically for the supression of PVCs. Procainamide is preferred over procaine as an alternative to lidocaine, when the latter has not been effective in suppressing PVCs or ventricular tachycardia. Like lidocaine, these drugs can not be relied upon to give pharmacologic defibrillation, but are used rather to enhance the chances of successful electric countershock. In the presence of spontaneous circulation they are more likely than lidocaine to produce hypotension. The recommended dose of procainamide is about the same as that of lidocaine. Repeat injections or infusion of procainamide must be stopped when the dysrhythmia has been controlled, or if hypotension occurs, or the QRS of the EKG is widened, or when a cumulative dose of about 1 gram of the drug has been reached. *Quinidine* is for long-term use.

Bretylium (Bretylol)

This is a new anti-dysrhythmic agent that raises the ventricular fibrillation threshold, probably through a post-ganglionic adrenergic blockade preceded by catecholamine release (Koch-Weser). This quarternary ammonium compound is presently recommended as a third line of defense in the control of ventricular tachycardia or ventricular fibrillation, when countershocks and lidocaine and/or procainamide have not been effective. It seems to facilitate subsequent electric defibrillation and prevent recurrent ventricular tachycardia or ventricular fibrillation in patients with very sick hearts. A variety of side effects associated with chronic administration, including postural hypotension and nausea, are irrelevant during the emergency use of this drug. Recommended doses are 5 mg/kg I.V. during CPR in recurrent ventricular fibrillation, followed by countershock. If ineffective in 5-15 minutes, a dose of 10 mg/kg is recommended, which may be repeated until a total dose of 30 mg/kg has been given. Continuous infusions of 1-2 mg/min have also been used. Bretylium is presently considered the ultimate drug when others have failed in the treatment of intractable ventricular tachycardia or ventricular fibrillation. In ventricular fibrillation, the *defibrillation threshold* is lowered (energy requirement reduced) by bretylium and clofilium (a new antidysrhythmic drug), but seems to be raised by lidocaine and quinidine (Babbs). For dilantin, see lit.

Propranolol (Inderal)

This beta-receptor blocker has no place in emergency resuscitation during cardiac compressions, as it may make the heart unresuscitable. Its principal use is in the patient with a spontaneous circulation accompanied by recurrent PVCs, ventricular tachycardia or atrial tachydysrhythmias, particularly when these dysrhythmias are triggered by pheochromocytoma, thyrotoxicosis or excessive amounts of beta-receptor stimulating drugs. Propranolol is used in a bolus of up to 1 mg/70 kg I.V. every 5 minutes, to a maximal dose of 5 mg. It is contraindicated in asthmatics and patients with myocardial failure.

Atropine

This is the classical parasympatholytic drug, which reduces vagal tone, enhances atrioventricular conduction, and reduces the likelihood of ventricular fibrillation triggered by the myocardial hypoperfusion associated with extreme bradycardia. It may increase the heart rate not only in sinus bradycardia but also in high degree atrioventricular block with bradycardia, but not in complete atrioventricular block, where isoproterenol is indicated. Atropine therefore has essentially no place during CPR Phases I and II, except possibly in refractory asystole

(Brown). During spontaneous circulation, however, when the heart rate decreases to less than about 50 beats per minute or there is bradycardia with PVCs or hypotension, atropine is indicated.

Atropine should be given in doses adequate to increase the heart rate, namely 0.5 mg/70 kg I.V., repeated as needed up to a total dose of about 2 mg, which results in complete vagal blockade. In third degree atrioventricular block larger doses may be tried although a beneficial effect is unlikely. Doses smaller than 0.5 mg/70 kg of atropine may lead to severe bradycardia which in the sick heart can trigger ventricular fibrillation; the heart rate is slowed probably via a central vagal stimulus or a peripheral parasympathomimetic action. In myocardial infarction or ischemia, tachycardia may increase the extent of infarct and even lead to ventricular tachycardia or ventricular fibrillation. Thus, atropine should be used with caution in such cases. It may be needed to counteract the bradycardia induced by morphine given for pain in acute myocardial infarction.

Digitalis

A variety of digitalis glycosides are in use today for their sustained positive inotropic effect (increase in the force of myocardial contraction), such as digoxin, lanatoside, and strophantin. Digitalis is also used to reduce the heart rate in atrial fibrillation. The value of digitalis in resuscitation is limited, since other drugs are more potent cardiovascular stimulants and have a wider margin of safety and faster action. Digitalis toxicity, combined with potassium depletion (e.g., from diuretics), should also be considered as a possible etiology for intractable dysrhythmias in patients undergoing resuscitation.

Nitroprusside

This rapidly acting peripheral vasodilating agent has no role during cardiac arrest and cardiac compressions. However, it has become a valuable adjunct for the reduction of peripheral vascular resistance and venodilation in protracted myocardial failure (to increase cardiac output) and for the control of hypertensive crises (Palmer). It does not affect cardiac rate and rhythm directly, although it may, through induction of hypotension, lead to reflex tachycardia. In myocardial ischemia with pump failure, even minimal reduction in peripheral arterial resistance by nitroprusside can sometimes bring cardiac output toward normal, enhance systolic emptying, relieve pulmonary congestion, decrease myocardial oxygen consumption and preserve ischemic myocardium. It should be given by infusion pump or microdrip, in a concentration of 50 mg/250-1000 ml, with pressure monitoring by intra-arterial and possibly pulmonary artery catheters (the latter optional). The pulmonary artery wedge pressure should be maintained at or above 15 mm Hg. The rapid and short action of nitroprusside calls for a carefully regulated infusion. The solution must be wrapped in aluminium foil as the drug deteriorates with exposure to light. The total dose should not exceed 100 mg per hour lest cyanide intoxication occurs.

Nitroglycerin

This classic direct vasodilator, used for the relief of angina pain, is now being used also for the reduction of preload and afterload by peripheral venous and arterial dilation, and for «internal phlebotomy» — in protracted cardiac failure — as an alternative to nitroprusside. The suggested I.V. solution is 50 mg/250 ml. For the acute relief of angina pain one nitroglycerin tablet of 1 mg administered sublingually, repeated up to 3 times at 3-5 minute intervals, has been recommended. Nitroglycerin tablets have also been administered sublingually in the emergency prehospital situation when treating acute pulmonary edema, where titrated infusions are not always feasible. Nitroglycerin has essentially no role during cardiac compressions.

Morphine

This ancient analgesic is not indicated during and immediately following CPR, but is one of several adjunctive drugs indicated in acute pulmonary edema, which may occur before or after cardiac arrest. Morphine seems to act by dilating capacitance vessels. producing a «bloodless (pharmacologic) phlebotomy», as well as reducing left ventricular afterload (Alderman). It may also improve pulmonary edema by relieving anxiety and depressing exaggerated breathing movements. In addition, morphine is an effective analgesic for the pain of acute myocardial infarction. The drug is best titrated I.V. by repeated individual doses of 2-5 mg/70 kg every 5-30 minutes, until the desired effect is reached. If it induces nausea or hypotension, a different analgesic, such as meperidine (Demerol, pethidine) or fentanyl should be substituted. With any narcotic, titrated administration must guard against hypotension and respiratory depression. Narcotics are contraindicated in spontaneously breathing patients with post-anoxic central nervous system depression. In the presence of controlled ventilation, however, any narcotic may be used liberally for analgesia and comfort of the intubated patient. With ventilation and blood pressure controlled, narcotics per se exert no deleterious effects on the brain. In some countries (e.g., Great Britain), heroin is available and then becomes the drug of choice for maximal analgesia and euphoria; its dose is 50% that of morphine.

Diuretics

Furosemide (Fousemide, Lasix) (0.5-2 mg/kg I.V.) ethacrynic acid (Edecrin) (0.5-1 mg/kg I.V.) inhibit the reabsorption of sodium in the loop of Henle. Furosemide has an additional veno-dilating effect. Diuresis starts within 5 minutes after I.V. administration, peaks at about one-half hour and lasts for several hours. The diuretic action of these drugs is indicated in pulmonary edema. Furosemide and ethacrynic acid may also reduce intracranial hypertension caused by post-anoxic or post-traumatic cerebral edema, partly because of a reduction in CSF production and increase in CSF clearance; and therefore in the post-arrest period at least one dose is usually indicated, provided normovolemia has been established.

Corticosteroids

These drugs may be used for their anti-inflammatory and anti-edema effects in the immediate post-resuscitative period, to ameliorate the reaction of the lungs to aspiration (which is common in CPR cases) and perhaps to reduce post-ischemic-hypoxic cerebral edema. Their value in shock and non-cardiogenic pulmonary edema is controversial. Suggested mechanisms by which corticosteroids act include stabilization of lysosomal membranes, prevention of histamine release, vasodilation, and protection of capillary integrity. Side effects associated with prolonged steroid medication, including reduced wound healing, reduced resistance to infection, stress ulcers, osteoporosis and adrenal cortical insufficiency, have not been proved to occur with short-term (3-7 days) use of pharmacologic doses of steroid, or with one massive dose. Large pharmacologic doses of corticosteroids have been recommended for cerebral edema, aspiration, or status asthmaticus: i.e., methylprednisolone 1 mg/kg (or dexamethasone 0.2 ml/kg) I.V., repeated every 6 hours up to 48 hours, and then gradually tapered over 1-2 weeks. For septic shock a single massive dose of methylprednisolone (5-30 mg/kg I.V.) is recommended. Steroid may be worth trying acutely as an adjunct in intractable electro-mechanical dissociation (White).

Miscellaneous Drugs

The physician should be familiar with the pharmacologic actions of the above mentioned drugs and in addition those drugs listed below for inclusion in the emergency kit. The induction of immobilization and apnea for stabilization of the comatose patient after cardiac arrest requires advanced respiratory care life support measures. Relaxants should be used only be professionals trained in anesthesia.

Physician's Emergency Drug Kit

1 **Epinephrine (adrenalin)**
2 **Sodium bicarbonate**
3 **Vasopressors**
   a. **Norepinephrine**
   b. **Metaraminol**
4 **Cardiotonics**
   a. **Isoproterenol**
   b. **Dopamine**
5 **Calcium chloride**
6 **Lidocaine; procainamide; bretylium**
7 **Propranolol**
8 **Atropine**
9 **Nitroprusside or nitroglycerin for infusion**

a. Nitroglycerin tablets
10 Morphine or meperidine (Demerol, pethidine)
11 Furosemide or ethacrynic acid
12 Methylprednisolone or dexamethasone
13 50 % dextrose (for empiric use in coma of unknown etiology)
14 Bronchodilators
   a. Aminophylline for I.V. infusion
   b. Metaproterenol for aerosol (a beta-2 receptor stimulator)
15 Diphenhydramine (Benadryl), an antihistaminic
16 Naloxone (Narcan) a narcotic antagonist
17 Barbiturate, short-acting (pentobarbital) or ultra-short-acting (thiopental)
18 Diazepam (valium); and diphenylhydantain (phenytoin)
19 Chlorpromazine (thorazine) as vasodilator, and for psychiatric emergencies
20 Muscle relaxant: succinylcholine (Anectine, suxamethonium) and pancuronium (Pavulon). Note: should be administered only by those experienced in their use. Produces apnea!
21 Mannitol (see Chapter III)
22 I.V. fluids (see subsequently)

Comment: In using drugs for emergency resuscitation, familiarity with the particular agent and therefore its skillful use, is more important than small differences in pharmacologic action between similarly acting agents. Not every «new» drug gives better results.

Fluids
Infusion Strategies, Hypovolemic Shock
During emergency resuscitation and post-resuscitative life support, I.V. fluids should be administered with the following objectives in mind:
1 To restore normal circulating blood volume immediately after fluid losses, using combinations of elctrolytes, colloids and red blood cell containing solutions (see below). Rapid, massive infusion of isotonic salt or colloid solutions can be life saving, particularly in cases of severe external or internal blood loss.
2 To expand normal circulating blood volume after cardiac arrest by about 10 % of estimated blood volume (10 ml/kg) in order to reverse the relative loss of blood volume brought about by vasodilation, venous pooling and capillary leakage.
3 To keep an I.V. route open for drug administration and at the same time provide basic hydration and glucose requirements. This may be accomplished by a continuous infusion of 5 per cent dextrose in 0.25-0.5 % sodium chloride, 20—25 ml/kg/24 hours for adults and children; 100 ml/kg/24 hours for infants. 5 % dextrose in *water* should *not* be used, as it may augment cerebral edema.

4 To adjust as soon as possible the above therapy for increased or decreased diuresis, keeping urine flow over 25 ml/70 kg per hour.
5 To modify I.V. fluids for optimal blood composition in terms of normal electrolyte concentrations, osmolality and colloid osmotic pressure; serum albumin $(3-5$ grams/dl); hematocrit $(30-40\%)$; and serum glucose $(100-300$ mg/dl).
6 To meet special requirements, such as osmotherapy in the early post-arrest period (see Chapter III) and artificial alimentation (dextrose, amino acids, vitamins) in the late post-arrest period.

In hypovolemic shock without cardiac arrest or in the post-cardiac arrest period, monitoring of arterial pressure, urine flow and CVP is needed for guiding volume replacement. CVP is a measure of the adequacy of right heart filling and function. The heart rate is also an indicator of the adequacy of circulating blood volume but less reliable. In addition, EKG and blood gases should be monitored when feasible. Overinfusion can be detected from a sustained rise in CVP; pulmonary rales or rhonchi (via esophageal stethoscope if the patient's trachea is intubated); or a decrease in arterial PO_2 with unchanged FIO_2 of $50\% - 100\%$ (indication of shunting).

For the rapid administration of large amounts of I.V. fluids, a short large-bore cannula and pressure infusion equipment are needed. Doubling the height of the infusion bottle doubles the flow rate, but doubling the internal diameter of the venous cannula increases the flow rate by 16 times. For the transfusion of blood or blood cells, micropore filters are recommended.

The amount and rate of I.V. infusion depend on the amount and rate of estimated blood volume loss and the type of fluid selected. Circulating blood volume (plasma plus red cell volume) normally accounts for $7-8$ percent of body weight (the figure 10% is used to simplify calculations). In a fit person, acute loss of up to about 10% of blood volume $(500-1000$ ml/70 kg) is mild hemorrhage and usually can be survived without therapy. Loss of about $10-20\%$ of blood volume $(1000-1500$ ml/70 kg) is moderate hemorrhage, which in most cases results in a picture of shock. Loss of $20-50\%$ of blood volume $(1500-3000$ ml) is severe hemorrhage, which always results in severe shock and, in most cases of over 30% blood volume loss, in irreversible shock and death if untreated. Finally, *rapid* loss of 40% or more of blood volume can rapidly lead to exsanguination cardiac arrest.

Extra-cellular fluid volume is normally about 25% of body weight in liters. It includes the intravascular space, i.e., plasma volume (5% of body weight) and the interstitial space (20% of body weight). Electrolyte solutions (isotonic saline, Ringer's solution) distribute throughout the entire extra-cellular fluid space — both intravascular and interstitial — and therefore electrolyte solutions should first be given in 4 times the quantity of blood volume lost. It is apparent that if moderate to severe blood loss is corrected by electrolyte solutions only, the creation of tissue edema is inevitable. Colloid solutions (blood, plasma, albumin, dextran, gelatin, starch), however, remain longer in the intravascular space (unless there is gross membrane leakage, as after very severe ischemic anoxia) and should therefore be given first in volumes equal to the blood volume lost.

When a *shock state* persists after replacement of estimated blood loss, after cardiac arrest without blood loss, or even following acute myocardial infarction, the hemodynamic state can benefit from incremental blood volume expansion with continuous monitoring of arterial pressure and CVP (and, optionally, pulmonary artery wedge pressure when left ventricular failure or shock lung is suspected). In the average adult, about 200 ml of electrolyte or colloid solution should be given rapidly I.V., and repeated every 10 minutes until the transiently increased CVP or pulmonary artery wedge pressure does not return toward normal, but rather remains higher than 3 mm Hg above the previous value (Weil).

When hemorrhage is being treated concurrently to prevent development of a shock state, moderate deliberate normovolemic *hemodilution* with plasma substitutes is a safe and sound practice in most previously healthy individuals. Hemodilution reduces blood viscosity and thereby improves blood flow and oxygen delivery to tissues, despite the reduced arterial oxygen content, at least down to a hematocrit of about 25% (Takaori, Messmer). The previously healthy organism can compensate with increased cardiac output for acute normovolemic anemia to a hematocrit of 25%; it can even survive a reduction in hematocrit to 10%, although with temporary decompensation (Takaori). The end point of useful hemodilution (uncompensated acute anemia) may, however, be above a 25% hematocrit in patients with cardiopulmonary disease. In any patient, this end point can be recognized by monitoring several parameters: blood base deficit will increase due to anaerobiosis and increased lactic acid (Fig. 35); furthermore, when the point of excessive hemodilution is reached, central venous PO_2 (normal value 40 mm Hg), decreases when oxygen transport does not keep up with oxygen demand. During hemodilution an FIO_2 of 100% is desirable, as an arterial PO_2 of 600 mm Hg can add 1.5 ml of oxygen (0.3 ml of oxygen per 100 mm Hg PO_2) to 100 ml of blood significant in shock or anemia.

Choice of I.V. Fluids

The choice of the optimal intravenous fluid for resuscitation remains controversial. Nonetheless, it is clear that replacing all blood loss with blood is neither sound nor necessary (Blalock). Blood can transmit hepatitis and can cause hemolytic reactions due to incompatibility.

Moreover typing and cross-matching delays availability of blood. Type-specific cross-matched fresh blood would be ideal, but often is not immediately available and is expensive. Stored, banked blood is also expensive, and entails additional risks, particularly in massive transfusions. These risks include hypothermia (cold blood leading to cardiac arrest), clotting factors deficiency, high potassium ion concentration, low pH, and microemboli. In general, safe blood and blood product services are expensive and may not be available in all regions of the world. Thus, the first line of therapy in blood loss and for blood volume expansion is I.V. infusion of a plasma substitute without red blood cells.

In moderate hemorrhage not exceeding 20% of blood volume, an *electrolyte solution* alone, such as isotonic sodium chloride (0.9%), or Ringer's solution, is adequate to maintain blood volume and homeostatis. As noted above, an electrolyte solution should be given in up to 4 times the blood volume lost, and more added to compensate for urine loss. Lactated Ringer's solution, which is only slightly less acid than Ringer's solution, and balanced salt solutions with normal pH (e.g., Normosol), are theoretically more physiologic than 0.9% sodium chloride solution. The latter, however, is cheaper and equally effective in treating moderate extracellular fluid loss.

In severe hemorrhage (over 20% of blood volume lost) use of electrolyte solutions alone is unphysiologic, as it produces tissue edema and is often incapable of maintaining blood volume, cardiac output and tissue oxygenation, even in 4:1 replacement volumes. In these cases a colloid plasma substitute should be given, at least for 1:1 replacement of volume lost beyond 20% of blood volume (Brinkmeyer, Thompson).

The choice of colloid plasma substitute is controversial. The normal colloid osmotic pressure of 25 mm Hg is maintained primarily by a serum albumin concentration of 5g/dl. A reduction of serum albumin concentration to one-half of normal reduces colloid osmotic pressure by two-thirds to the level at which tissue edema tends to develop. Human serum *albumin* 5% in isotonic saline, or commercial plasma *protein fractions* (e.g., Plasmanate), which contain mainly albumin plus a small amount of globulins, are sterile and safe. They are ideal colloid plasma substitutes. However, they are very expensive and often unnecessary, since serum albumin and globulin levels are fairly rapidly restored from body pools. Therefore, *dextrans, gelatin, starch* solutions or other adequately tested synthetic colloids are also recommended. These products are inexpensive and suitable for long-term storage, and they support survival as well as albumin and better than salt solutions (Gelin, Takaori, Shoemaker). Dextran 70, 6% in isotonic saline, has a 30% intravascular retention after 24 hours; Dextran 40, 10% in isotonic saline, has a shorter retention, but reduces sedimentation rate and may have a more potent anti-sludging effect. Dextran 40 should, however, be given only after urine flow has been restarted with electrolyte solutions, since it tends to plug renal tubules. Hydroxyethyl starch, 6 % in isotonic saline, has characteristics similar to Dextran 70. It should be noted that all plasma substitutes, electrolyte and colloid solutions, produce hypocoagulability by diluting the clotting factors. Dextrans and starches, in addition, coat platelets, thus adding further to the anticoagulant effect. Although dextrans have caused anaphylactic reactions, allergic reactions are rare and unimportant for emergency resuscitation; no such anaphylactic reactions have so far been reported with hydroxyethyl starch. Synthetic colloids may interfere with typing and crossmatching of blood (therefore draw blood first), unless a cell washing laboratory technique is used.

Plasma pooled from multiple donors may transmit hepatitis. Pasteurized plasma preparations (e.g., 5 % plasma protein fraction) are safe, except when occasionally found to contain vasodilator substances. Fresh frozen plasma is indicated in certain hemorrhagic diatheses.

Banked blood or *packed red blood cells* should be used to sustain the hematocrit at or above 25 to 30 %. In the absence of hematocrit determinations, whole blood or red cells (if available) should be added to plasma substitutes, when estimated blood loss reaches and exceeds 30 % of blood volume, or the patient was anemic prior to hemorrhage. The preservative-anticoagulant CPD, citric-acid-phosphate-dextrose has replaced ACD, citric-acid-citrate-dextrose.

During massive infusions of banked blood or red cells, calcium administration is usually not needed; but blood should be warmed to near body temperature on the way into the patient. Sodium bicarbonate should be given to correct measured base deficit. To prevent coagulation problems, it has been suggested to add fresh frozen plasma (250 ml/70 kg) for every 1/2 blood volume (2500 ml/70 kg) of stored blood infused.

Packed red blood cell solutions, because of their high hematocrit, need dilution with isotonic saline solution added to the bag, to enhance flow rate in the infusion for hemorrhage. Undiluted packed red cells are recommended in anemia associated with heart failure or hypertension.

The physician charged with responsibility for resuscitation should be familiar with coagulation problems caused by protracted shock states and massive blood transfusions; he should be conversant with the simple clotting tests available for bedside use and with the indications for certain blood components and heparin. Such therapies are beyond the scope of this manual.

Oxygen carrying blood substitutes, such as *stromafree hemoglobin* (Amberson) and *fluorocarbons* (Geyer), are presently under clinical investigation. They may soon influence the treatment of massive blood loss. Unfortunately stromafree hemoglobin is rapidly lost from the circulation, and fluorocarbons may have effects on tissues in which they are stored long-term, which effects are still unclear. The fluorocarbon solution Fluosol DA 20 % (Naito) presently under clinical trials, requires high FIO_2 and carries less oxygen than hemoglobin, but more than plasma substitutes. The latter, however, promote blood flow better.

Emergency resuscitation for hypovolemic shock is required not only in cases of trauma, hemorrhage and burns, but also in cases of severe *diarrhea* (e.g., cholera). In the extra-hospital treatment of mass outbreaks of diarrheal disease, or treatment of traumatic shock in conscious victims of mass disasters, when I.V. fluid administration is not possible, *oral fluids* have a place in the treatment of mild to moderate hypovolemic shock. Commercially available oral replacement powders, when diluted as recommended, yield isotonic or one-half isotonic Ringer's solution plus carbohydrates, vitamins, amino acids, and flavoring to give them an acceptable taste. The Red Cross recommends to add 1 teaspoon of sodium chloride and 1/2 teaspoon of sodium bicarbonate to each liter of water to be taken by mouth. However, fluids must never be given by mouth when the patient is stuporous or comatose, because of risk of aspiration.

ELECTROCARDIOGRAPHIC DIAGNOSIS

Techniques of Electrocardiography
As soon as possible after the start of CPR-ABC, the electrocardiographic (EKG) pattern should be determined, primarily to differentiate between: (1) ventricular fibrillation (or ventricular tachycardia with coma); (2) electric asystole; and (3) pulselessness (mechanical asystole) with bizarre EKG complexes, also called «electromechanical dissociation» or «cardio-vascular collapse» (Fig. 36). These are the three most common patterns associated with the clinical picture of cardiac arrest (pulselessness of carotid and femoral arteries). Epinephrine and sodium bicarbonate are indicated in all three conditions. In addition, ventricular fibrillation and ventricular tachycardia call for immediate electric countershock, the only reliable means of defibrillation.

The EKG is not an indicator of circulation. Even normal EKG complexes can continue for many minutes in the presence of mechanical asystole. Thus, during resuscitation, monitoring of the EKG is important, but only adjunctive to palpation of the carotid, femoral, and peripheral pulses; monitoring arterial pressure (by Riva-Rocci cuff technique and, as feasible, by arterial catheter); and examining skin and mucous membranes for color, temperature and capillary refill. In the patient with endotracheal tube in place, an esophageal stethoscope is also recommended, as it is the simplest, cheapest and most reliable device for monitoring breathing and circulation. It permits hearing each heart beat and assessing the strength of cardiac contractions; it also enables clear audition of breath sounds, which give a clue about tidal volume, bronchospasm and secretions. The esophageal stethoscope is not recommended for use during cardiac compressions. Ideally an endotracheal tube should be inserted first, the gastric tube next, and the esophageal stethoscope last. All this may be possible only after restoration of spontaneous circulation.

The *techniques* for EKG pattern display during emergency resuscitation have been greatly simplified by the fact that modern defibrillator paddles incorporate the EKG pick-up electrodes. This permits instantaneous recognition of ventricular tachycardia or ventricular fibrillation and immediate countershock therapy.

During CPR, EKG monitoring should be initiated as soon as possible with a method that does not hamper cardiac compressions and artificial ventilation. This is best done by the application of the electrodes to the extremities. For Lead II, the negative electrode is usually placed on the right arm, the positive electrode on the left leg, and the indifferent electrode on the left arm. Use of needle electrodes fastened with tape provide a more rapid and more secure EKG than disc electrodes fastened with rubber bands or stick-on electrodes.

Long-term EKG monitoring during the Phase III of CPR calls for a replacement of the extremity electrodes to the chest, so that they do not limit limb motion or interfere with periodic 12 lead EKGs, which might be needed later to diagnose myocardial ischemia. For Lead II by chest electrode, place the negative electrode just below the right clavicle, the positive electrode below the left pectoral muscle, and the indifferent electrode anywhere, for instance just below the left clavicle. For modified Lead V-1, which is the best lead for distinguishing between right and left ventricular ectopic activity as well as for detecting and recording atrial activity, place the positive electrode over the right fifth intercostal space and the negative electrode over the left shoulder (outer third of the left clavicle); the ground electrode is usually most comfortably attached near the right shoulder (outer third of the right clavicle).

EKG Monitoring in Resuscitation

1 Establish an airway; begin artificial ventilation and external cardiac compressions.
2 Apply quick-look defibrillation paddles to patient's chest for rapid EKG diagnosis. If ventricular tachycardia or coarse ventricular fibrillation is seen, give immediate countershock. (Cardiac compressions must be interrupted for a few seconds to permit accurate diagnosis).
3 During prolonged CPR-ABC, apply needle or stick-on electrodes to patient's extremities. Lead II: right arm (negative electrode), left leg

(positive electrode), left arm (ground).

4 After restoration of spontaneous circulation, when perfusion is stable, switch from extremity electrodes to stick-on chest electrodes. Lead II, V-5: right clavicle (negative), left fifth interspace (cardiac apex) (positive), left clacivle (ground).

5 Lead V-1: left clavicle (negative), right fifth interspace (positive), right clavicle (ground). Lead V-1 is preferred for recognition of PVCs.

The radio-transmission of EKG patterns (EKG telemetry) has been useful for the prevention of cardiac arrest by early recognition of life-threatening dysrhythmias in ambulatory hospitalized patients; and for prehospital emergency cardiac care, when paramedics in the field are under physician direction by radio. The latter, however, does not require EKG telemetry if the paramedics are trained in pattern recognition.

Since most sudden cardiac deaths associated with myocardial ischemia or infarction occur following life-threatening dysrhythmias, EKG monitoring should be used as a *preventive measure* in all patients with suspected myocardial infarction or shock. Cardiac arrest can often be prevented by early detection.

EKG Patterns of Cardiac Arrest (Fig. 36, 38)

Ventricular fibrillation is the most common cause of sudden cardiac death. It is an irregular, continuous, peristaltic, quivering motion of the ventricles of the heart that does not pump blood and that is associated with the characteristic EKG pattern of oscillations without intermittent ventricular complexes. Ventricular fibrillation may be primary or secondary, but in any case its mechanism is still not entirely clear. Ventricular fibrillation is most often due to spotty areas of hypoperfusion of the myocardium (transient, focal myocardial ischemia, sometimes as a result of vasospasm, sludging, or hypotension) in either sick hearts or in «hearts too good to die» (Beck). The latter are capable of producing adequate cardiac output once ventricular fibrillation is reversed.

Asystole can be mechanical asystole plus electrical asystole (pulselessness with cardiac standstill and isoelectric EKG) or mechanical asystole (pulselessness) with the isoelectric EKG intermittently interrupted by ineffective normal or abnormal EKG complexes at regular or irregular intervals. Asystole may be primary or secondary. Most commonly it is caused by hypoxia, asphyxia, exsanguination or heart block. Before accepting a persistently isoelectric EKG as asystole, «disguised ventricular fibrillation» should be ruled out by checking the EKG with a second electrode position, 90° to the first.

Electromechanical dissociation is mechanical asystole (pulselessness) with agonal (bizarre, abnormal) or relatively normal EKG patterns (see asystole). This condition has in the past also been labeled «cardiovascular collapse». There are no characteristic QRS patterns.

All three EKG patterns mentioned above (shown in Fig. 36) are incompatible with life, since they do not produce any blood flow.

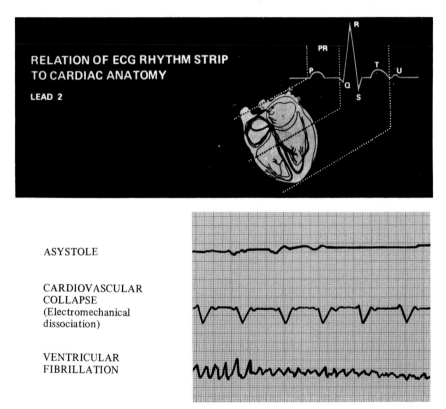

Figure 36: Electrocardiographic diagnosis of cardiac arrest

Top: Relation of normal EKG to cardiac anatomy.

Bottom: The three typical EKG patterns associated with pulselessness — (1) asystole; (2) electromechanical dissociation (cardiovascular collapse, mechanical without electrical asystole); and (3) ventricular fibrillation. Electromechanical dissociation is not associated with a characteristic QRS pattern.

(From American Heart Assoc. Dallas TX USA)

Life-Threatening Dysrhythmias (Fig. 37—39)

Health professionals providing advanced CPR life-support must be able to recognize at least the following tachy- and brady-dysrhythmias:

Premature atrial contractions are *not* life-threatening and are usually harmless; they may occur in normal persons. If they are frequent, they may indicate heart disease and initiate atrial tachycardia. They are important primarily because they need to be distinguished from PVC's which *are* sometimes dangerous. Therapy for premature atrial contractions consists of sedation,treatment of the underlying problem if any (Greenbaum) and interdiction of coffee and cigarettes.

Atrial fibrillation can also appear occasionally in normal hearts, but is more likely a sign of heart disease. It results in an irregularly irregular ventricular rhythm, which is the hallmark of this dysrhythmia and makes it immediately recognizable even on palpation of the pulse. Atrial fibrillation is not life-threatening unless associated with a very rapid ventricular rate. It is usually treated first by digitalis. If unsuccessful, the most effective treatment is synchronized electric (low energy) DC countershock (cardioversion); but this should be undertaken with great caution in the digitalized patient. Propranolol may also have a place in the treatment of atrial fibrillation with a rapid ventricular response, especially when the clinical situation permits a more leisurely therapeutic approach.

Premature ventricular contractions (PVCs) (Fig. 37) are usually bizarre extra EKG complexes triggered by an ectopic focus. PVCs can be felt as extra pulse beats. Often PVCs do not produce a pulse because of inadequate ventricular filling. The PVC is followed by a compensatory pause, which the patient can sometimes feel as a momentary «fullness» in the chest. Frequent multifocal PVCs are the most common *precursors* of ventricular tachycardia and *ventricular fibrillation* (i.e., sudden cardiac death), and a PVC falling on a T-wave (R-on-T phenomenon) very often initiates ventricular fibrillation. More than 6 PVCs in a row are by definition called ventricular tachycardia. If every other beat is preceded by a PVC, it is called «ventricular bigeminal rhythm»; if it is every third beat, it is called «trigeminal rhythm». Single PVCs of similar configuration that do not fall on the T-wave occur in healthy persons and may be harmless; in ischemic hearts, however, they also may represent an increased risk.

PVCs are treated with an I.V. bolus of lidocaine (1 mg/kg), followed by a lidocaine infusion (1—4 mg/minute per 70 kg). Later, long-term preventive medication may include procainamide, diphenylhydantoin, propranolol, quinidine, digitalis, or other drugs. In very slow heart rates, such as in heart block (see below), PVCs may represent an «escape rhythm» and can be prevented by the use of atropine, isoproterenol, or pacing. However, atropine and isoproterenol in themselves may result in tachydysrhythmias.

Ventricular tachycardia (Fig. 37) is the most dangerous precursor of *ventricular fibrillation* (Fig. 38). Ventricular tachycardia is a regular sequence of bizarre runs of PVCs. During ventricular tachycardia there may or may not be a palpable pulse, depending in part on the rapidity of the rate. When there is a pulse, and the patient is conscious, lidocaine should be administered I.V. in an attempt to terminate ventricular tachycardia; however, ventricular tachycardia with unconsciousness or pulselessness must be treated immediately like ventricular fibrillation, namely with electric countershock and CPR as needed.

It is important to differentiate between ventricular and supra-ventricular tachycardia, since the latter is not immediately harmful and the former is life-threatening. If the differentiation is impossible, the hemodynamic effects of the dysrhythmia, as monitored by pulse, arterial pressure and CVP, should guide therapy. Eventually, even *atrial tachycardia* should be treated, particularly in the elderly with coronary artery disease (Valsalva maneuver, carotid sinus massage, methoxamine, verapamil, digitalis).

Figure 37: EKG patterns of tachydysrhythmias (All lead II).
(1) One PVC with R-on-T, causing ventricular fibrillation (VF) (no pulse). (2) Occasional unifocal PVCs (possibly harmless). (3) Frequent multifocal PVCs (dangerous). (4) PVCs causing ventricular tachycardia (can be short run, terminating spontaneously). (5) Sustained ventricular tachycardia.
(Adapted from American Heart Assoc. Dallas TX USA)

Bradycardia (Fig. 39) is defined as a heart rate of less than 60 per minute. It is dangerous in the critically ill person when the heart rate is less than 50—60 per minute, irrespective of whether it is sinus bradycardia or bradycardia of ventricular origin. One should always make an attempt to differentiate between these two. Sinus bradycardia is harmless in healthy persons and common in athletes; but can be risky in patients with myocardial disease. Bradycardia of ventricular origin is life-threatening as it is due to a block in the cardiac conduction system.

Atrioventricular block may be first, second or third degree. *First degree* A-V block is merely a delayed passage of the impulse through the A-V node, causing a prolonged P-R interval. It serves as a warning, but rarely is treatment needed. *Second degree* A-V block results in dropped beats and may be one of two types — the Mobitz type I pattern (Wenckebach A-V block) and the more dangerous Mobitz type II pattern. Mobitz type I A-V block is common in myocardial infarction, usually transient, and if associated with significant bradycardia requires atropine or isoproterenol rather than a pacemaker. In inferior wall myocardial infarction, Mobitz type I block may precede Mobitz type II A-V block, which occurs in large myocardial infarctions, often as a forerunner to complete A-V block. The appearance of Mobitz type II AV block indicates the need for at least a standby pacemaker.

Figure 37

(1) PVC with R-on-T
   resulting in
   ventricular fibrillation

(2) PVCs

(3) Multifocal PVCs

(4) PVCs with
   Ventricular
   Tachycardia

(5) Ventricular
   Tachycardia

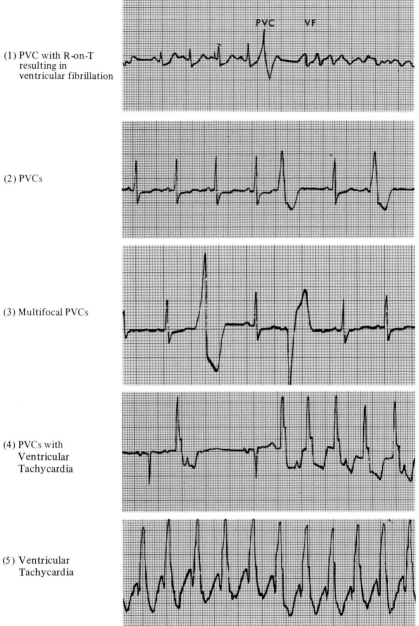

Figure 38

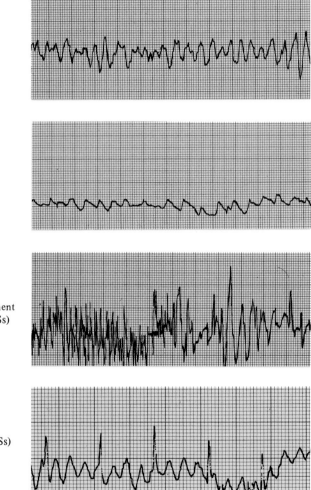

(1) Coarse
Ventricular
Fibrillation

(2) Fine
Ventricular
Fibrillation

(3) Artifact,
patient movement
(includes QRSs)

(4) Atrial flutter
(includes QRSs)

Figure 38: EKG fibrillation patterns

(1) Coarse ventricular fibrillation (pulselessness). (2) Fine ventricular fibrillation (pulselessness). (3) Artifact from patient movement, with QRS complexes and with pulse. (4) Atrial flutter, with QRS complexes and with pulse.

(From American Heart Assoc. Dallas TX USA)

Figure 39:

(1) First degree AV block
     (prolonged
     P-R interval)

(2) Second degree AV block
     (Mobitz I, Wenckebach)

(3) Second degree AV block
     (Mobitz II) 2:1

(4) Complete AV block

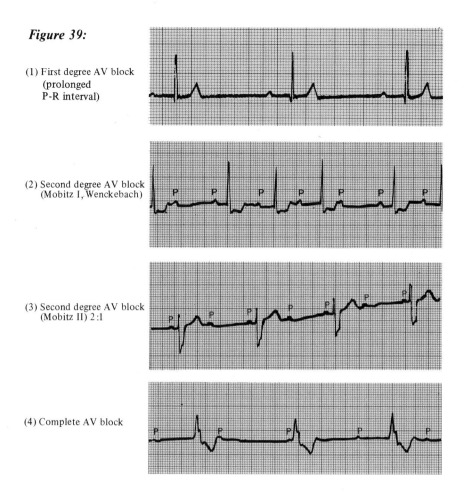

Figure 39: EKG patterns of bradydysrhythmias (All lead II).
(1) First degree AV block (fixed prolonged P-R interval). (2) Second degree AV block (Mobitz type I-Wenckebach phenomenon) (expanding P-R interval). (3) Second degree AV block (Mobitz type II) i.e., 2:1 block, evolved from (2). (4) Complete AV block with ventricular rhythm. In (3) and (4) a pacemaker is indicated.
(Modified from American Heart Assoc. Dallas TX USA)

Third degree (complete) A-V block is characterized by an absence of conduction of impulses from the atria to the ventricle, with a slow idioventricular rate of 30 to 40 beats per minutes, as in Stokes-Adams syndrome. The P-waves are unrelated to the QRS complexes. With a very slow ventricular rate, blood flow may become inadequate to maintain consciousness, and reduced myocardial perfusion can result in congestive heart failure, angina, ventricular tachycardia or ventricular fibrillation. Treatment in the patient who tends to become unconscious or whose heart rate is considered dangerously slow, should consist of external «first pacing» while an I.V. infusion of isoproterenol is started. With this treatment the patient's heart rate usually can be supported adequately until an I.V. pacemaker is inserted. During CPR-ABC, when upon restoration of spontaneous circulation there are recurring runs of ventricular tachycardia or even ventricular fibrillation, one should study the EKG in detail to determine whether the tachydysrhythmia is preceded by third degree (complete) A-V block. In this instance *lidocaine is contraindicated,* and seemingly paradoxic treatment with isoproterenol and pacing may keep the sinus rate high enough to prevent such recurrent ventricular tachydysrhythmias and cardiac arrest.

In general, atropine is more effective for increasing the heart rate in sinus bradycardia than in ventricular bradycardia (complete heart block), when isoproterenol is more effective. Patients with acute myocardial infarction of the anterior wall (which carries a high mortality) can suddenly develop complete heart block and are usually unresponsive to atropine. In contrast, patients with acute myocardial infarction of the inferior wall (which carries a low mortality) can develop bradycardia due to increased vagal tone with a slow progression to Mobitz II block and finally to third degree atrieventricular block; these sometimes do respond to atropine.

Dysrhythmias with pulselessness call for immediate resuscitative action. Dysrhythmias with a palpable pulse and consciousness call for thoughtful assessment and *treatment of the whole patient,* not merely the EKG!

FIBRILLATION TREATMENT (Defibrillation) (Fig. 40)

Electric defibrillation is indicated for the termination of the lethal dysrhythmias of ventricular tachycardia (with coma or without pulse) and ventricular fibrillation. Primary causes of ventricular fibrillation include coronary insufficiency, adverse drug reactions, electrocution, cardiac catheterization in an irritable heart; ventricular fibrillation may also occur secondarily, during resuscitative efforts for asystole from asphyxia, drowning, exsanguination, and other causes of cardiac arrest. While appropriate drug therapy can often *prevent* ventricular fibrillation, drug treatment cannot by itself be relied upon to *terminate* ventricular fibrillation. Lidocaine, quinidine, potassium chloride and beta-blockers usually cannot in the absence of countershock terminate ventricular fibrillation, but may instead transform ventricular fibrillation into asystole that is subsequently intractable to CPR efforts, including epinephrine.

The most rapid, effective and accepted method for terminating ventricular fibrillation is *electric countershock* (Prevost, Beck, Gurvitch, Peleska, Zoll, Lown). Spontaneous cessation of ventricular fibrillation without countershock is very rare in man, although common in small animals. *Low* voltage electric shock, which sends less than 2 amperes through the heart (e.g., electrocution by electric house current) can induce ventricular fibrillation. Properly applied *high* voltage electric shock, which sends more than 2 amperes through the heart produces in the normally beating heart a sustained contraction (e.g., shock by lightning), and can terminate ventricular fibrillation (e.g., therapeutic countershock of 500 volts alternating current (AC) or 300 joules direct current (DC) across the chest) (Hooker, Kouwenhoven). Such defibrillating shocks produce simultaneous depolarization off all myocardial fibers, after which spontaneous cardiac contractions may start *if the myocardium is well oxygenated and non-acidotic.* The amount of current actually passing through the heart cannot be monitored, but delivered energy can and should be monitored.

Techniques for electric countershock that minimize chest wall resistance and optimize electric shock wave patterns, durations, delivered voltage in AC shock, and delivered energy (watt-seconds or joules) in DC shock, have evolved empirically. DC rather than AC countershock is more effective in enlarged, diseased hearts, as well as in hypothermic patients and for cardioversion. The DC shocks' short duration and ability to be programmed exactly in cardioversion can prevent application of the electric shock on the upstroke of the T-wave of the EKG, which can induce ventricular fibrillation in the beating heart of the victim. Also the operator is endangered if he is not protected by insulation. In the treatment of ventricular tachycardia and ventricular fibrillation this advantage of DC over AC countershock is irrelevant. However, even in

131

defibrillation, AC countershock has no advantages and some disadvantages over DC countershock: AC defibrillators depend on wall current, thus are not portable; muscle contractions are strong; the longer impulse required can cause ventricular fibrillation in the spontaneously beating heart; and there is an additional hazard to the operator because of non-isolated current flow.

EKG diagnosis and electric countershock must go hand in hand. To produce the required energy in the heart, an *AC countershock* (now obsolete) usually of 500 to 1000 volts (0.1 to 0.25 second), applied directly to the outside of the chest is required in the average adult. Although lower voltage shocks may sometimes succeed, higher energy levels are recommended because failure of the first countershock may delay restarting of spontaneous circulation.

The same applies to the presently used *DC countershock,* which has the added advantage of being superior for cardioversion in the beating heart. DC countershock is produced by a capacitance discharge-type defibrillator, delivering up to 400 watt seconds (Joules) in about 0.01 second duration. Although subtle histologic changes in the myocardium are related to the amount and duration of current transmitted through the heart, and, thereby, to the heat produced in the myocardium, external application of such high energy or high voltage countershocks does not cause enough damage to impair resumption of spontaneous contractions. This risk of producing heat damage may be greater when low voltage or low energy is used frequently, as in the case when the first defibrillation attempt with inadequate energy fails. Also, recovery of the brain is enhanced by immediate restoration of spontaneous circulation. In contrast, direct application of high energy shocks to the heart during open chest CPR can produce burns on the surface of the heart.

Although the most commonly used energy for external DC countershock is 400 watt seconds for adults, 100 to 200 Joules for children, and 50 to 100 Joules for infants, lower energies occasionally have been effective in ventricular tachycardia and sometimes even in ventricular fibrillation. However, the ideal amount of energy required in any given case cannot be determined during CPR in advance. While the above energy recommendations are for the conventional single discharge wave form, other wave forms may have different energy requirements. For this the manufacturer's literature should be consulted.

Defibrillators must be checked frequently to determine the actual energy delivered, since the reading on the dial is not always accurate. A regular maintenance program for defibrillators is essential. Defibrillators should be tested at low and high levels and should be capable of delivering up to 400 watt seconds (Joules) DC (Nobel).

Chest defibrillating *paddles* for external defibrillation should be large for optimal propagation of current, i.e., 14 cm diameter for adults, 8 cm for older children, and 4.5 cm for infants. Paddles for open chest (internal) direct application on the heart should have diameters of 6 cm for adults, 4 cm for children and 2 cm for infants.

The present recommended *technique* of *external* countershock is as follows (Babbs, Tacker, American Heart Association) (Fig. 40):

In witnessed arrest apply countershock within 30–60 seconds of the onset of ventricular fibrillation. In unwitnessed arrest apply CPR-ABC for about 2 minutes before an initial attempt to defibrillate.

Have a helper set up and charge the DC defibrillator (probably a portable unit). (If using an AC defibrillator, have him plug it into the wall outlet). Have the helper ready to hand you the two paddles. Good electric contact between electrodes and skin is essential, but electrode paste should not be used so liberally that it produces a current path between electrodes over the patient's skin. Electrode paste makes the chest slippery for external cardiac compressions whereas saline-soaked sponges do not. The sponges have the added advantage of being applied more rapidly, so minimizing interruption of CPR, but again they should not be so soaked that saline oozes between the defibrillator paddles. Apply just enough electrode paste on the defibrillator paddles or apply saline-soaked sponges on the patient's chest (do not use both). Request an assistant to charge the defibrillator. Apply the two standard defibrillator paddles to their appropriate positions, namely the negative (black) paddle just to the right of the upper half of the sternum below the clavicle, and the positive (red) paddle just to the left of the cardiac apex or below the left nipple. Press the two paddles firmly over the sponges to the chest in the appropriate locations. Press hard to force exhalation, as this decreases thoracic impedence.

Read the EKG as picked up by the defibrillating chest paddles and ascertain ventricular tachycardia or ventricular fibrillation before triggering the shock. When ready, ask the team to stand clear of patient and bed for the moment of shock.

Know in advance which type of cardioscope-defibrillator is in your service. Some cardioscopes are protected, but others must be disconnected prior to countershock, lest they be damaged.

The defibrillator should have been preset for 200-300 Joules energy for the *first countershock* in an adult. The suggested initial energy dose for external countershock is 3 Joules per kg for adults and 2 Joules per kg for children. The highest repeat dose is 5 J/kg.

Discharge the countershock by pushing the appropriate hand switches, (preferably one on each paddle to avoid accidental discharge).

The defibrillator shock is best applied by the individual who directs the team. A convulsive motion will be caused by the skeletal muscle stimulation by electric shock. Immediately after this countershock remove the paddles, oberserve the EKG and resume IPPV and cardiac compressions, and repeat the procedure if indicated.

After successful defibrillation, the EKG may show asystole, abnormal EKG complexes, or approximately normal EKG complexes. Irrespective of what the EKG monitor shows, cardiac compressions must be continued so long as there is no spontaneous carotid or femoral pulse. If the EKG shows asystole, CPR, epinephrine and bicarbonate must be continued.

If ventricular fibrillation persists or recurs after the first 2 electric countershocks, with $200 - 300$ watt seconds (70 kg adult), you should *repeat countershocks* several times, as needed, up to *360 watt seconds* in adults, i.e. 5 watt seconds per kg, with CPR in between. If several maximal energy (360 watt seconds) countershocks fail to terminate ventricular fibrillation in spite of optimal cardiac compressions and IPPV, and reasonable amounts of epinephrine and bicarbonate, give lidocaine 1 mg/kg I.V. Repeat lidocaine if necessary. Efforts to reverse ventricular fibrillation with appropriate drug therapy (including bretylium) and repeated high energy countershocks, should be continued until successful, or until irreversible asystole occurs with signs of myocardial death (intractable electric asystole).

Do not give up attempts to defibrillate until efforts have been made to improve acid-base status, oxygenation and vasoconstriction by epinephrine. Some patients have recovered consciousness after defibrillation following several hours of ventricular fibrillation, during which time cardiac compressions produced borderline circulation. Such cases however are rare.

In witnessed, monitored ventricular fibrillation, apply external countershock immediately, without first giving drugs or starting CPR-ABC. If unsuccessful, start CPR promptly to minimize cerebral and myocardial hypoxia, administer drugs and repeat the electric countershocks. Adapt the sequence of actions according to parameters monitored and the patient's underlying condition. Countershock is more likely to be successful if given one-half to two minutes following the I.V. administration of epinephrine during CPR. Do not wait with countershock until the large volume of sodium bicarbonate has been injected.

When several individual countershocks fail to terminate ventricular fibrillation, repeat several (serial) shocks in rapid sequence. Rapid serial defibrillation attempts were easily accomplished using the AC defibrillator, which does not require recharging; but considerable pauses are needed between shocks with the DC defibrillator, because it requires a few seconds to recharge. Thus cardiac compressions will have to be interposed between serial countershocks with a DC defibrillator.

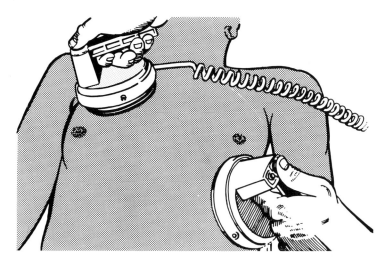

Figure 40: External electric defibrillation via two bimanually triggered chest paddles applied on conductive jelly or saline-soaked sponge, one paddle just below right clavicle, the other over the cardiac apex. The paddles incorporate defibrillation outlets and EKG leads.

Technique of External Electric Countershock

1 CPR-ABCs ongoing. (In sudden witnessed arrest defibrillate within 30 seconds without CPR-ABC).
2 Turn synchronize switch of defibrillator *off.* Turn main power switch *on.*
3 Set energy level to desired reading (approx. 3 Joules/kg).
4 Charge the paddles.
5 Lubricate the paddles with electrode paste. Interrupt the rescuer's chest compressions as briefly as possible (15-20 seconds maximum) for countershock. Place paddles on chest. Negative paddle — just to the right of the upper sternum, below the right clavicle. Positive paddle — just below and to the left of the left nipple
6 Apply firm pressure with the paddles against the chest.
7 Confirm EKG diagnosis.
8 Clear the area.
9 Fire the defibrillator. (Prefer defibrillators with switches on both handles of paddles).
10 Leave paddles in place 5 seconds to ascertain rhythm.
11 If a pulse is not palpable within 5 seconds, resume CPR-ABCs.
12 If VF continues after 1 min. CPR, repeat countershocks with 3 . . . 4 . . . 5 Joules/kg.

In the absence of a cardioscope and the presence of a defibrillator (which is rare) it is quite justifiable to use an *empirical (unmonitored) DC countershock* for witnessed cardiac arrest. Electric countershock does not do any further damage in asystole or electromechanical dissociation; although it is not effective in restarting the heart in these conditions. Such a single shock, however, should not delay the start of other CPR measures. Unmonitored countershock in children is not recommended. Countershock without EKG diagnosis is rarely necessary, because of the increasing availability of EKG monitors combined with defibrillators.

Experimental semi-invasive defibrillation techniques, using *esophageal*-to-chest surface electrodes, reduce the electric resistance between electrodes and therefore the total energy required; this may enable development of a very small portable defibrillator (Elam). *Automatic implantable defibrillators are under clinical trials (Mirowski).*

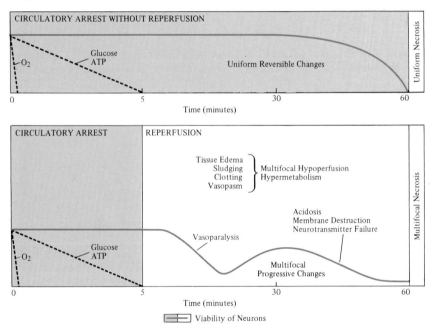

Figure 41: Diagram of hypothetical events following circulatory arrest. Without reperfusion (top), brain damage becomes clearly irreversible (necrosis) only after 30 to 60 minutes of arrest. With reperfusion after periods of arrest longer than 5 minutes (bottom), secondary changes are provoked, which, added to the initial insult, result in multi-focal necrosis. Brain resuscitation research seeks to ameliorate these secondary changes and thereby help recovery of neurons (from Safar P: Hospital Practice 16:67, 1981).

PROLONGED LIFE SUPPORT

Post-Resuscitative Brain-Oriented Therapy

Chapter III

Phase III of CPCR (Fig. 1) is long-term resuscitation, that is intensive care life support for multiple organ failure. It consists of a combination of Steps «G» (Gauging, i.e., evaluation and critical care triage); «H» (humanizing the outcome by brain resuscitian measures); and «I» (intensive therapy for general life support). These measures require considerable medical judgment and skills. All 3 steps should be taught and applied simultaneously, since long-term life support after emergency resuscitation (Step I) (Table IV) should be brain-oriented (Step H) (Tables V, VI) and applied with reason; the latter entails estimation of the severity of the insult (Table VII), evaluation of early predictive criteria (most of which are still under investigation) of long-term outcome (Table VIII), and criteria and methods for discontinuing resuscitation efforts (Tables IX, X).

INTENSIVE THERAPY WITH CEREBRAL RESUSCITATION

The socio-economic impact of brain injury secondary to cardiac arrest, stroke, other anoxic states, and cerebral trauma is enormous, and this impact falls in varying degrees upon the sufferer, upon his family and upon society. The patient's outcome in terms of survival and overall performance capability (particularly human mentation) depends on the severity and duration of the insult, the speed and quality of emergency resuscitation, and the early start and high quality of brain-oriented, post-resuscitative intensive therapy. While such post-resuscitative treatment cannot alter the initial insult, it has been shown to influence *secondary changes* that occur in all vital organ systems after the start of reperfusion and reoxygenation, i.e., the «post-resuscitation disease» (Negovsky). The most important component of this post-resuscitation disease is multi-focal impaired reperfusion of the brain (Ames, Nemoto, Plum). Some cerebral neurons can recover after 30-60 min. of circulatory arrest (Hossmann).

The failure of one organ system influences the function of others, and there is no doubt that the failure of extra-cranial organ systems influences the brain. For example, hypotension, hypoxemia, hypercarbia, severe hypertension, hyperthermia, struggling, pain, «stress», coughing, sepsis, renal failure, and other severe extra-cerebral alterations have all been shown to add to the initial insult, worsen cerebral edema and ischemia, and worsen the neurologic deficit (Blayaert, Safar). Even without these complications, however, global ischemia with reperfusion after 5-7 minutes, results in multi-focal brain necrosis (Moosy). Reperfusion provokes transient vasoparalysis; spotty hypermetabolism; tissue acidosis; release of free chemical radicals that tend to damage membranes; and varying degrees of intra- and extracellular edema (Siesjo). Probably all vital organ systems suffer from changes post-CPR (Negovski, Gurvitch).

The objectives of «post-resuscitative brain-oriented intensive therapy» are:
1 To optimize respiratory, cardiovascular, metabolic, renal and hepatic function for survival of the entire organism;
2 To apply these measures in a way which will benefit particularly the recovery of cerebral neurons (standard, non-controversial measures of brain-oriented life support); and
3 To investigate in patients the benefits and risks of additional special (novel) brain resuscitation measures, most of which are still experimental and controversial.

The guidelines of Table IV are for the conscious or unconscious patient; those of Tables V and VI are for the comatose patient. These guidelines are by no means sacrosanct; they merely serve as check lists for patient management, which should be adapted according to the patient's underlying disease and available resources and intensive therapy services (Kucher and Steinbereithner; Lawin; Ledingham; Safar and Grenvik; Schwartz; Safar et al; Shoemaker and Thompson; Weil).

Respiratory and Cardiovascular Support (Table IV)
After cardiac arrest of several minutes' duration and subsequent restoration of spontaneous circulation, the patient usually suffers from multiple organ failure for hours or days. This post-arrest syndrome of multiple organ failure usually includes protracted acidosis and reduced cardiac output, as well as occasional disseminated intravascular coagulation and «self-poisoning» from renal and hepatic failure. The situation may be complicated by aspiration syndrome, flail chest from sternal compressions, acute pulmonary edema, or progressive pulmonary consolidation (i.e., adult respiratory distress syndrome, shock lung). The latter may be due to prolonged hypoperfusion, trauma or sepsis. Respiratory failure after cardiac arrest and CPR should be managed with the measures described in Chapters IA and IB (Pontoppidan, Safar, Smith J.).

Cardiovascular support after CPR must aim at prevention and treatment of life-threatening dysrhythmias and shock states. *Shock* is the clinical picture of overall inadequate tissue perfusion and oxygenation.

TABLE IV

Respiratory and Cardiovascular Support
Prevention and Treatment of Shock and its Complications

I. Immediate measures

Prevent hypoperfusion (blood volume, pump, pressure) — (Chs IC, II).
Maintain and optimize art. press., CVP, urine flow, EKG, temperature
   Maintain and optimize pulm. art. (mean and wedge) pressures (as indicated); keep COP — PAWP over 5 mm Hg.
   Maintain urine flow over 25 ml/70 kg/hr
   For IV fluids, see Chapter II
Maintain and optimize art. PO_2, PCO_2, pH, base excess — (Chs IA, IB).
   FIO_2 100%, to 50% as soon as possible
   Controlled or intermittent mandatory ventilation
   Optimize PEEP (effective compliance, central venous PO_2)

II. Urgent measures

Chest X-rays; sputum examination
Aseptic airway and catheter care
Drain stomach; drain pus; drain hematoma
Control fluid intake and output; monitor body weight
Monitor and optimize blood hematocrit, sugar, cell count, clotting variables
Maintain and optimize plasma colloid osmotic pressure
Maintain and optimize serum and urine osmolality
Maintain and optimize serum electrolytes, proteins

III. Additional measures

Diuresis; (hemodialysis)
5 % albumin I.V.(test the effect of 200 ml challenges on PaO_2, CVP, PAWP)
Alimentation (IV or gastrointestinal tube) 2,000-4,000 calories/24 hrs/70 kg (Dextrose 10-20%, amino acids, vitamins, essential fatty acids)
Steroid (?); Dextran 40 (?); Heparin (?)
Correct the underlying problem

Shock states may be divided into: (1) Hypovolemic (oligemic); (2) cardiogenic (pump failure); (3) obstructive (pulmonary embolism, cardiac tamponade); or (4) distributive (e.g., septic shock) (Shubin). An aggressive approach to the prevention or immediate reversal of shock states is aimed at the prevention of secondary post-resuscitative deterioration to «irreversible shock» and re-arrest, and also at the prevention of acute renal failure, progressive pulmonary consolidation and fat embolism syndrome after multitrauma. Methods for managing shock are described in Chapter II and further detailed in Table IV (Weil, Shoemaker, Cowley).

Standard Measures of Brain-oriented Life Support (Table V)
There are several accepted measures, based on experimental evidence or extensive clinical experience, that are useful after a severe ischemic-anoxic insult for supporting recovery of neurons. These measures are for extra-cranial homeostasis, i.e., to control extracerebral organ systems function in ways which would benefit the brain (Table V-A); and for intracranial homeostasis, particularly control of intracranial pressure (ICP) (Table V-B) (Grenvik, Safar, Shapiro, Snyder, Trubuhovich).

The *extracranial homeostasis* measures for the comatose patient (Table V-A 1-10) start with control of arterial blood pressure, to avoid both any degree of hypotension (defined in terms of the individual patient) as well as severe hypertension. After cardiac arrest, normotension or mild sustained hypertension may be beneficial. (After head trauma, normotension or mild hypotension is to be preferred). After cardiac arrest, immediately upon restoration of spontaneous circulation, a brief period of hypertension (which usually occurs as the result of epinephrine given during CPR) may help overcome initial sludging and stasis in the microcirculation (Hossmann). Tracheal intubation and mechanically controlled ventilation, if necessary with partial neuromuscular blockade utilizing a curarelike agent such as pancuronium (Pavulon), allow for prolonged immobilization, which facilitates control of arterial pressure and blood gases, and thereby may reduce the severity of brain injury (Bleyaert, Safar). Avoidance of fully paralyzing doses of the relaxant enables recognition of awakening and of hemiplegia. Noxious afferent stimuli should be eliminated. Treatment or prevention of restlessness, straining, and more serious events such as seizures, may require a central nervous system depressant, such as intravenous thiopental (Pentothal) or pentobarbital (Nembutal) in conventional anesthetic doses that do not depress the cardiovascular system. Other alternatives for deafferentation and control of seizures are use of diphenylhydantoin (Dilantin, phenytoin), diazepam (Valium) or etomidate.

The provisions of moderate controlled hyperventilation (better by mechanical ventilation than by the patient himself), aiming at an arterial PCO_2 of 25 to 35 mmHg, is recommended to counteract cerebral acidosis, to decrease ICP by decreasing intracranial blood volume, and to perhaps shift blood flow inside the damaged brain from reactive healthy areas to damaged areas with absent blood flow autoregulation. The arterial PO_2 should be maintained over 100 mmHg with the highest inhaled oxygen concentration considered safe (50% long-term), and avoidance of mean airway pressure higher than necessary (minimal PEEP). The arterial pH should be maintained between 7.3 and 7.6. The value of the early use of a corticosteroid following cardiac arrest has not been documented, but since adjunctive benefits cannot be ruled out and short-term use of steroids is safe, they are included in the protocol for optional use.

Maintenance of optimal hematocrit, electrolytes, plasma colloid osmotic pressure, serum osmolality, blood sugar, hydration and alimentation (Manni) must be assured.   Normothermia should be maintained; hyperthermia must be avoided.

The *intracranial homeostasis* measures (Table V-B, 1-5) start with the ruling out of an intracranial mass lesion which would require immediate operation. Unwitnessed asphyxia or cardiac arrest are sometimes the result of acute intracranial hematoma (e.g., post-trauma). Even in the patient under the influence of a relaxant or an anesthetic, a mass lesion can be suspected from the history and from unilateral mydriasis, and proven by CAT scanning or cerebral angiography.

Intracranial pressure (ICP) monitoring has become increasingly common for guiding interventions to control ICP. After moderate global ischemic-anoxic insults (cardiac arrest), cerebral edema is rarely severe enough to increase ICP. However, if there is initial neurologic improvement, followed (usually on the second day) by secondary deterioration, ICP may rise and should be monitored where facilities for safe, atraumatic, aseptic ICP monitoring are well established. The hollow skull screw (Becker) is favored in medical coma, but is technically sometimes unsatisfactory. The ventricular catheter (Lundberg) is favored after head trauma. Both methods carry infection risks. Trials of new epidural pressure probes appear promising. ICP monitoring is more often indicated in coma after head injury or encephalitis than after cardiac arrest.

The monitored increases in ICP above the desired level of 15 mmHg or less (zeroed at level of mid-cranium) are used to guide titrated stepwise measures for *ICP reduction* (Table V-B, 2): further hyperventilation ventricular cerebro-spinal fluid drainage; osmotic diurectics such as mannitol; loop diurectics (e.g., furosemide); an intravenous anesthetic such as thiopental; glucocorticoid therapy; and hypothermia (see «Special Measures for Brain Resuscitation»).

While short-term (12 to 48 hours) low-dose osmotherapy with mannitol or glycerol continues to be utilized, intracranial hypertension is increasingly controlled with anesthetic doses of intravenous thiopental or

TABLE V

Standard Measures of Brain-Oriented Life Support
Guidelines for coma following global ischemia-anoxia

A. **Extracranial homeostasis**

1 Control mean arterial pressure (MAP); normalize blood volume

Plasma volume expansion (e.g., 10 ml/kg); vasopressor/-vasodilator

(a) Brief mild hypertension (MAP 120-140 mm Hg) for 1-5 min immediately after restoration of circulation (optional)

(b) *Maintain normotension* (MAP 90 mm Hg) or slight hypertension (MAP 100-120 mm Hg) throughout coma (Note: After cerebral trauma maintain normotension or slight hypotension, MAP 60-90 mm Hg)

(c) Vascular catheters — arterial and central venous catheters; pulmonary artery balloon catheter (optional)

2 Immobilization with softening doses of relaxant (e.g., pancuronium), if necessary for controlled ventilation.

3 Drugs IV for deafferentation (analgesia-anesthesia) and prevention/control of seizures; e.g., thiopental or pentobarbital 5 mg/kg IV plus 2 mg/kg per hr (plasma level 2-4 mg/dl), total 30 mg/kg (more for recurrent seizures); or diphenylhydantoin (Dilantin, phenytoin) 7 mg/kg IV, repeat prn, or diazepam (Valium), or etomidate.

4 Arterial PCO_2 25-35 mm Hg, by controlled ventilation

5 Arterial pH 7.3-7.6

6 Arterial PO_2 over 100 mm Hg, with FIO_2 50% and minimal PEEP

7 Corticosteroid (optional): methylprednisolone 5 mg/kg IV followed by 1 mg/kg per 6 hrs IV; or dexamethasone 1 mg/kg IV followed by 0.2 mg/kg per 6 hrs IV; short-term (2-5 days)

8 Blood variables:

Hematocrit 30-35%; electrolytes normal

Plasma colloid osmotic pressure over 15 torr (albumin over 3 g/dl)

Serum osmolality 280-330 mOsm/liter

Glucose 100-300 mg/dl

9 Maintain normothermia; avoid hyperthermia

TABLE V (continued)

   10 Fluids: No Dextrose in water only.
Use Dextrose 5-10% in 0.25-0.5% NaCl IV,
30-50 ml/kg per 24 hrs (100 ml/kg per 24 hrs in infants);
add potassium as needed

   11 Alimentation: Dextr. 20 %, aminoacid, electol, vitamins

B. Intracranial homeostasis

   1 Rule out mass lesion (history, clinical picture; cerebral angiography or CAT scanning in selected cases)

   2 *Monitor* intracranial pressure (only if safe technique established) — optional after CPR; recommended after head injury and in encephalitis —

     (a) hollow skull screw (Becker) preferred in non-traumatic coma

     (b) ventricular catheter (Lundberg) preferred in traumatic coma

     Control intracranial pressure at or below 15 mm Hg by:

     (a) further hyperventilation ($PaCO_2$ to 20 mm Hg)

     (b) ventricular CSF drainage

     (c) Mannitol 0.5 g/kg IV; plus 0.3 g/kg IV per hr, short-term. (Optional: mannitol 1g/kg once IV, empirical. without ICP monitoring, immediately following restoration of spontaneous circulation after cardiac arrest), repeat when neurologic deterioration

     (d) loop diuretic IV (e.g., furosemide 0.5-1.0 mg/kg IV)

     (e) thiopental or pentobarbital 2-5 mg/kg IV, repeated as needed (this table A-3)

     (f) corticosteroid (this table A-7)

     (g) hypothermia, 30-32°C, short-term (with controlled ventilation, relaxant, anesthetic, vasodilator) short-term hypothermia optional; long-term hypothermia not recommended

   3 Monitoring of electroencephalogram (optional)

     (a) regular EEG

     (b) computerized EEG (cerebral function monitor)

     (c) evoked potentials (experimental)

     (d) treat EEG seizures (this table A-2,3)

   4 Additional experimental measurements — cerebral electric impedance, cerebral blood flow and metabolism, cerebrospinal fluid composition (see text)

   5 Evaluate insult (Table VII); depth of coma (coma scoring); and long-term outcome (Table VIII)

pentobarbital, particularly when the need for treatment extends for more than 24 hours or when large doses of osmotic agents are required for ICP control. In this last circumstance, rebound edema and severe disturbance of blood volume-, fluid -, and electrolyte balance may be major complications of osmotherapy, and thus limit its usefulness.

It should be noted that although the ICP controlling measures listed above were developed from experience with patients after brain surgery or head injury, these measures are also appropriate for selected comatose patients with encephalitis, severe stroke or after cardiac arrest. ICP monitoring also assists in detecting circumstances that may inadvertently increase ICP (e.g., tracheal suctioning, change of body position).

Other advanced measures for promoting intracranial homeostasis, most of which are still experimental, include EEG analysis and recording of evoked EEG potentials (technically difficult in the ICU setting); measurements of cerebral blood flow and metabolism, which would require sampling of cerebral venous (superior jugular bulb) blood; measurement of cerebral electric impedance; and analysis of CSF for pH (normal value 7.3), lactate (normal value 1.5-2 micromoles/ml, 14-18 mg/dl), cyclic AMP and enzymes (CPK, GOT, LDH) (Mullie). Evaluating insult and outcome , as well as neurologic signs early after the insult, which might permit prediction of outcome (see later), should be part of standard management of the comatose patient after emergency resuscitation.

Special Measures for Brain Resuscitation (Table VI, Fig. 41)
The potential importance of experimental evidence for effective treatment of post-ischemic-anoxic encephalopathy is obvious. Most of the special brain resuscitation measures to be discussed here are new or under re-investigation, and still controversial. Confusion and controversy have arisen because of incautious conclusions drawn from comparisons of experimental results with different animal models, treatment and post-insult management. One must keep in mind the differences between the kinds of injury produced in the brain by ischemia, anoxia, hypoglycemia, anemia, trauma, hemorrhage, metabolic or toxic abnormalities, inflammation, or by different combinations of these processes. With ischemic insults, there are as well important distinctions between global ischemia, as in shock states or cardiac arrest, and the focal ischemia of cerebral infarction. There are also differences between reduced blood flow, as in shock, and total cessation of flow, as in cardiac arrest. Finally, in considering therapeutic measures, one must differentiate between *protection,* i.e. measures instituted before an insult, and *resuscitation,* i.e., measures taken after an insult.

Presently available evidence of the efficacy of some promising specific brain resuscitation measures is presented in Table VI. The clinician may *promote reperfusion* by providing immediately and during the first few hours post-ischemia, moderate sustained hypertension (Nemoto) with vasopressor and plasma volume expansion, plus moderate normovolemic hemodilution to hct. 25-30 %, using a colloid plasma substitute (Jurkiewicz, Safar). At this time there is no proof that post-ischemic heparinization improves reperfusion or post-ischemic cerebral recovery (Safar); pre-insult heparinization (e.g., for cardiopulmonary bypass), however, might increase the brain's tolerance of ischemia (protection). Severe hypertension (MAP over 150 mm Hg) seems to be deleterious (Bleyaert).

Some of the measures which appear most promising in possibly saving neurons, if applied post-ischemia, are controversial because their possible benefit is accompanied by known risks. These measures include the use of anesthetics such as barbiturates, anticonvulsants, immobilization, osmotherapy and hypothermia (Table VI).

Barbiturates are known to reduce cerebral metabolic rate and edema formation and to suppress seizure activity, implying a protective influence on survival. There is also evidence to suggest that barbiturates exert a beneficial effect via anesthetic blockade of noxious stimuli. There are other possible mechanisms of barbiturate action that have not yet been fully documented, including the stabilization of membranes and altering metabolic pathways. Barbiturates seem to reduce intracranial blood volume and ICP; and can silence EEG activity.[*]

Large and moderate doses or thiopental and pentobarbital, given before or after experimental permanent focal ischemia (ischemic stroke), have been shown to reduce the size of the infarct (Smith A, Hoff). There have been beneficial results when barbiturates were given to animals before ischemia (protection) (Goldstein, Secher) or during hypoxia (Yatsu). In patients, the value of anesthetic doses of thiopental or pentobarbital to reduce ICP has been demonstrated (Shapiro). The presently only available evidence that barbiturate can save neurons when given *after total* circulatory arrest, is the report that thiopental loading (with doses large enough to possibly re-arrest the heart) after circulatory arrest to the head in monkeys, can reduce brain damage significantly (Bleyaert). This study has stimulated in recent years widespread interest in brain resuscitation research in general and in barbiturate therapy in particular. A prospective international clinical study of thiopental loading after cardiac arrest will yield results in 1983 (Safar). Its protocol calls for thiopental 30 mg/kg IV given as early as possible after cardiac arrest to patients who are comatose at 10-20 minutes after restoration of spontaneous circulation. Blood pressure is supported with plasma substitute and vasopressor. Feasibility trials on patients appeared promising (Breivik).

The clinician must bear in mind that the circulatory depressant effects of large doses of thiopental or pentobarbital are considerable, particularly in the patient with heart disease or hypovolemia, and that the

[*]With a thiopental or pentobarbital plasma level of 4 mg/dl (Gisvold).

risk/benefit ratios of this treatment versus conventional (safe) doses have not yet been determined. Optimal dosage, blood levels and timing of barbiturate administration are still unclear (Breivik, Gisvold).

In the meanwhile, conventional anesthetic doses of thiopental or pentobarbital (2-5 mg/kg IV, repeated as needed) that do not depress the circulation and require only small amounts of vasopressor and plasma volume expansion, may be clinically indicated to sedate, suppress seizures, facilitate controlled ventilation, reduce «brain stress» and normalize monitored rise in ICP. Even this less controversial treatment should be used early and by physicians skilled in the administration of these anesthetics, and only for patients who are comatose after severe global or focal ischemic-anoxic or other brain insults. Barbiturate anesthesia for protection against anticipated brain ischemia during neurosurgical and cardiothoracic surgical cases also seems justified. We do *not*, however, recommend the *routine* use of large loading doses of barbiturates at this time. All this is now (1981) in a state of flux.

After head injury or encephalitis, administration of prophylactic barbiturate, without ICP monitoring, is controversial. In shock states with coma, cardiovascular stabilization has therapeutic priority, since barbiturate may precipitate cardiac arrest in hypovolemia. And in that barbiturate suppresses neurologic function, and the usual clinical signs are depressed, careful diagnostic evaluation is necessary. Physicians and the public should be made aware of the fact that benefit can be expected from barbiturate therapy only if it is started immediately after the insult.

Barbiturates may not necessarily emerge as *the* therapeutic anesthetic to «put the injured brain to rest». Anticonvulsants like *diphenylhydantoin* (Dilantin, phenytoin) or anesthetics with cerebral metabolic depressant effects similar to those of barbiturates, which depress arterial pressure less than barbiturates, should also be studied.

Immobilization with a muscle relaxant for 48 hours post-ischemia ameliorated experimental post-ischemic brain damage (Bleyaert, Gisvold), perhaps because it facilitated control of extracerebral organ systems' variables. Early post-arrest immobilization is included in the standard protocol (Table V).

Osmotherapy given immediately after reperfusion has not yet been studied in controlled animal models. Its ability to ameliorate brain damage is suspected from its ability to reduce brain edema, but has not yet been documented (Table VI).

Therapeutic *hypothermia* after ischemic brain insults reduces the rate of brain metabolism, the magnitude of cerebral edema and the size of experimental infarcts (Rosomoff). The resuscitative effect of hypothermia after global ischemia has not yet been documented by controlled studies. Hypothermia has not gained wide acceptance because of the difficult management problems it entails, especially after 12-24 hours; it is also associated with a variety of undesirable injurious side effects, such as increased incidence of dysrhythmias, elevated blood viscosity with reduced blood flow, and increased susceptibility to infection and stress ulceration. Still, the protective effect of hypothermia induced before total circulatory arrest is unquestioned, its' resuscitative effect needs controlled study.

In patients with a previously healthy cardiovascular system (e.g., children after drowning) short-term moderate hypothermia is justified. One feasible technique is the reduction of body temperature to 30-32°C for 3-12 hours, as early as possible after the insult, followed by gradual rewarming to normothermia. To use hypothermia safely, the patient's defense reaction to cooling must be blocked, to induce poikilothermia. Therefore cooling must be accompanied by relaxation (using a neuromuscular blocking agent), controlled ventilation, and drugs to block (prevent) the hypothermia-induced shivering, hypermetabolism, vasoconstriction and dysrhythmias. All this can be accomplished by chlorpromazine (Thorazine), 5-10 mg slowly IV, repeated with titration as necessary (avoiding hypotension); or by anesthetics such as thiopental or pentobarbital. Using a barbiturate may add to the cerebral protecting

TABLE VI

Special Measures for Brain Resuscitation

(Evidence as of 1980)

Treatment	Cardiac arrest Animal	Man	Brain infarct Animal	Man	Cerebral Trauma Acute ICP rise Animal	Man
Moderate hypertension	(+)		(+)	(+)		
Hemodilution (iv)	(+)		+	(+)	(+)	
Heparinization	(+)		−	−	−	−
Severe hypertension	−				−	−
Thiopental-high-dose	+	*	+		+	+
Thiopental-conventional dose			+		+	+
Phenytoin (Dilantin)	(+)					
Immobilization, controlled hyperventilation	(+)		(+)			(+)
Osmotherapy			(+)		+	+
Hypothermia		(+)	+		(+)	+

− = may be harmful, (+) = possibly reduces brain damage, + = reduces brain damage, Blanks: not studied.
* Pittsburgh collaborative study, results 1983.

effect of hypothermia, Barbiturates, hypothermia and phenytoin all have different mechanisms of action (Michenfelder).

Other measures which might be beneficial in saving neurons post-arrest, based on past studies and clinical impressions, and which deserve investigation for use immediately post-arrest, include hypertonic glucose (with or without insulin and ATP); CSF pH normalization; and various anesthetics, sedatives, free radical scavengers and calcium blockers which do not depress the blood pressure. Any safe measure which minimizes brain metabolism, improves microcirculatory blood flow, reduces brain edema, normalizes brain pH, or stabilizes membranes deserves study first in the laboratory and then in patients. Volatile anesthetics such as halothane, which also reduce metabolism like barbiturates, may be harmful to the damaged brain, since they increase cerebral blood flow and ICP and depress blood flow autoregulation within the brain. «Therapeutic anesthesia» is not a new idea (Laborit).

In the near future, treatment for brain insults will probably not consist primarily of barbiturates, but rather will include some anesthetic as part of a combined pharmacological and physiological scheme of therapy. Post-ischemic, -hypoxic, and -traumatic encephalopathies have multifactorial pathogeneses; therefore effective brain resuscitation measures will have to be multifaceted. Physicians involved in resuscitation should remain informed about current developments in cerebral resuscitation.

EVALUATION AND CRITICAL CARE TRIAGE
Definitions of Death
Modern resuscitation has led to changes in the definition of death.

Clinical death is apnea (no spontaneous breathing movements) plus total circulatory (cardiac) arrest, with all cerebral activity suspended, but not irreversibly so. It is that early period of death during which initiation of resuscitation, provided therapy is optimal, might be followed by restoration of all vital organ systems function, including normal brain function.

Cerebral death (cortical death) is irreversible destruction (necrosis) of the cerebrum, particularly the neocortex; *brain death* (total brain death) is cerebral death plus necrosis of the rest of the brain, including cerebellum, midbrain and brain stem (Beecher). Cerebral death and brain death often become apparent following restoration of circulation by CPR, with or without initial transient improvement of neurologic status. Most patients who develop brain death after cardiac arrest do so within the first week. Most medical and legal authorities now define «death» in terms of brain death, even though the heart may still be beating and artificial ventilation is maintained.

Biological death (panorganic death) inevitably follows clinical death when there is no intervention with CPR or when resuscitation efforts are abandoned. Biological death is a necrotizing process of all tissues, starting with cerebral neurons, which become necrotic after about one hour without circulation; followed by heart, kidneys, lungs and liver, which become necrotic after about 2 hours without circulation; to the skin which does not become necrotic for many hours or days.

«Social death» (persistent vegetative state; appalic syndrome) represents irreversible severe brain damage in a patient who remains unconscious and unresponsive, but has an active electroencephalogram (EEG) and some intact reflexes. This is to be distinguished from cerebral death, in which the EEG is silent and from brain death, in which in addition all cranial nerve reflexes and spontaneous breathing efforts are absent. In vegetative state there can be wake-sleep cycles.

Evaluating («Gauging») (Tables VII, VIII)
This should include attempts to assess: (1) the severity of the insult; (2) prognostic criteria early post-insult, such as the state of consciousness and post-arrest cranial nerve reflexes; and (3) the ultimate long-term outcome in terms of the patient's performance capability and quality of life. Because of the scarcity of reliable data on resuscitation results, this author recommends ongoing evaluation of resuscitation services, using the simple methods developed recently at the University of Pittsburgh for a collaborative, international study of CPCR (Copy Tables VII and VIII for your use). See also Case Report Form (page 239).

Evaluation of the Insult (Table VII)
The severity and duration of the insult influences the outcome of the ischemic-anoxic brain injury, as do the adequacy of resuscitation, the underlying disease, and secondary complications. The severity of traumatic brain insult is in itself almost impossible to quantitate. However, the severity of a global ischemic-anoxic insult, like cardiac arrest, can be estimated immediately retrospectively from interviewing bystanders, relatives, ambulance personnel and other health care personnel. We recommend estimating «arrest time», «CPR time», «hypoxia times» and «total insult time» (Table VII).

Evaluation of Coma
The degree of unresponsiveness (depth of coma), at least so long as the patient is in the ICU after a cerebral insult, can and should be followed. This may be accomplished by one of the following two coma scales:
1 The Glasgow Coma Scale (Teasdale), which has become popular as an effective method of quantitating the depth of CNS depression. It uses a $3 \times 5 = 15$ point scale (coma with brain death = 3 points; conscious and neurologically normal = 15 points). This scale has been tested and used primarily for evaluation of patients with cerebral trauma.
2 The Glasgow-Pittsburgh Coma Scale, which is being used in a

TABLE VII

Estimation of Global Ischemic-Anoxic Insult

Pittsburgh Cardiac Arrest Form
1978

1 Hypoxia time prior to arrest
Time of severe hypotension, severe hypoxemia, or severe anemia ....min

2 Arrest time
Time without spontaneous or artificial pulse in large arteries. Must *not* include CPR time ....min

3 CPR time
Equals time of CPR-ABC, i.e. borderline perfusion by cardiac compressions ....min

4 Hypoxia time after arrest
Time of severe hypotension, severe hypoxemia, or severe anemia following restoration of spontaneous circulation ....min

5 Total insult time
Sum of (1), (2), (3) and (4) ....min

Repeated arrests and repeated restoration of spontaneous circulation within one resuscitation effort, should be stated as the sum of all times without circulation (total arrest time) and the sum of all times of hypotension, hypoxemia and anemia (one total hypoxia time), whether this occurred before, or after the first or subsequent arrest.

controlled clinical study (Safar, Detre). It imploys a 7 x 5 = 35 point scale (coma with brain death = usually 7 points; conscious and neurologically normal = 35 points). It was designed for evaluation of comatose patients after any type insult, including cardiac arrest. The Glasgow score can be extracted from the Pittsburgh score, which is still being field tested and is available from the author.

A coma score will be low if the patient is under the influence of CNS depressants or neuromuscular blockers. Thus it is preferable that the depth of coma following CPR be scored before the administration of CNS depressants or neuromuscular blocking drugs. It should then be repeated at 6 to 24 hour intervals, until recovery of consciousness.

When assessing the depth of coma, rapid recovery of eye and upper airway reflexes should be considered good prognostic signs. Poor (but not hopeless) prognostic signs, on the other hand, include absence of the oculocephalic (doll's eye) or oculovestibular (caloric) reflex at 6 to 12 hours post-arrest; continuing unconsciousness and non-reactivity of the pupils; and progressive deterioration of reflexes after initial partial recovery (Bates). Pupil size, eye and lid movements, EEG activity (difficult to reliably determine in the ICU setting) and return time of spontaneous breathing are less reliable as prognosticating indicators.

Evaluation of Outcome (Table VIII)

The outcome after emergency resuscitation, in terms of quality of life, as evident from patient performance capability should be evaluated. The Glasgow outcome Categories 1 (best) through 5 (worst) (Jennett, Bates) provides a simple mechanism for categorizing patients' performance capabilities after head injury. The Glasgow - Pittsburgh cerebral performance categories (CPC) and overall performance categories (OPC) separate cerebral form extra-cerebral disabilities (Table VIII). This is essential for the evaluation of the effect of new treatments on cerebral recovery, versus mortality and morbidity due to the underlying disease (most commonly cardiovascular failure). Each category should be assessed upon discharge from the ICU, and periodically thereafter up to one year. Of particular interest is the best cerebral performance category which the patient achieves post-resuscitation.

Briefly, the cerebral and overall performance categories are as follows (Table VIII): Category (1) means a normal status without disability; (2) means conscious with slight disability; (3) means conscious with severe disability; (4) means coma or vegetative state without brain death; and (5) is brain death. For example, a conscious, mentally active, bedridden, post-CPR patient with severe heart disease would have a cerebral performance category 1 and overall performance category 3. Differences in cerebral and overall performance categories are for (1), (2) and (3); while categories (4) and (5) are determined by the cerebral status only. Ideally, CPC and OPC should be followed at least 6 months.

When Not to Undertake Emergency Resuscitation

Resuscitation should not be undertaken when the patient is in the terminal stages of an incurable disease; when the physician's orders include «do not resuscitate» or «no CPR»; or when there is another acceptable reason to withhold CPR. Among such acceptable reasons are situations in which there is no reasonable chance to restore human mentation — e.g., when clinical death has progressed to the point of rigor mortis, evidence of tissue decomposition, or extreme dependent lividity — and of course, decapitation.

Uncertainty regarding the possibility of brain death should *not* deter resuscitative efforts, since brain death cannot be determined immediately, and newer techniques for post-arrest treatment show promise in mitigating the damaging effects of ischemia-anoxia on the brain.

TABLE VIII A

Cerebral and Overall Performance Categories

Glasgow-Pittsburgh
1978

(A) CEREBRAL PERFORMANCE CATEGORIES (CPC)
Evaluate only cerebral performance capabilities. Estimate *potential* performance if non-cerebral organ systems were (are) normal.

CPC 1. Good cerebral performance: Conscious, alert, able to work, might have mild neurologic or psychologic deficit.

CPC 2. Moderate cerebral disability: Conscious, sufficient cerebral function for independent activities of daily life. Able to work in sheltered environment.

CPC 3. Severe cerebral disability: Conscious, dependent on others for daily support because of impaired brain function. Ranges from ambulatory state to severe dementia or paralysis.

CPC 4. Coma or vegetative state: Any degree of coma without the presence of all brain death criteria. Unawareness, even if appears awake (vegetative state) without interaction with environment; may have spontaneous eye opening and sleep awake cycles. Cerebral unresponsiveness.

CPC 5. Brain death. Apnea, areflexia, EEG silence (see Table X).

CPC A Under the effect of anesthetic (CNS depressant or relaxant).

TABLE VIII B

(B) OVERALL PERFORMANCE CATEGORIES (OPC)
Reflects cerebral *plus* non-cerebral status.
Evaluate *actual* overall performance.

OPC 1. Good overall performance: Healthy, alert, capable of normal life, CPC 1.

OPC 2. Moderate overall disability: Conscious, CPC 2, or moderate disability from non-cerebral systems dysfunction alone, or both. Performs independent activities of daily life, but is disabled for competitive work.

OPC 3. Severe overall disability: Conscious, CPC 3, or severe disability from non-cerebral organ systems dysfunction alone, or both. Dependent on others for daily support.

OPC 4. Coma or vegetative state: Same as CPC 4.

OPC 5. Brain death: Same as CPC 5.

When to Terminate Emergency Resuscitation

In acute respiratory or circulatory distress, the medical professional or trained lay person on the spot must start resuscitation immediately. There is no time for contemplation or consultation. When, however, *after* the start of emergency resuscitation, it becomes known that the patient is in the terminal stage of an incurable disease, or that he is almost certainly incapable of regaining cerebral function (e.g., after one-half to one hour of proven pulselessness at normothermia without CPR), all the resuscitation efforts may be discontinued. The dicision to terminate resuscitation should, whenever possible, be made by a physician, who must use his own and his colleagues' experience and knowledge to guide his decision. Common sense must play a large role in determining when to stop resuscitation in any given case.

Cardiac death (irreversible cardiac arrest).
In all salvageable patients, CPR efforts should be continued until spontaneous circulation is restored or signs of cardiac death (irreversible cardiac arrest) are present. Cardiac death is evident when there has been intractable electric asystole (flat line on the EKG) for at least about 30 minutes, despite optimal CPR and drug therapy. Pulselessness in the

presence of EKG complexes (mechanical asystole without electrical asystole) is *not* proof of irreversibility. So long as EKG activity continues, one must assume that there is still a chance for restarting spontaneous circulation; and indeed, EKG activity may continue for many minutes after cardiac arrest without resuscitation, and for hours during CPR. During closed-chest CPR without EKG monitoring, irreversibility cannot be proven, since ventricular fibrillation may be present, and ventricular fibrillation is always potentially reversible. There have been cases of ventricular fibrillation with CPR of several hours duration, followed by successful defibrillation and recovery of consciousness.

Brain death.
It is impossible to judge the salvageability of the brain during emergency resuscitation. Therefore, cardiac death (plus apparent brain death) should be the criterion for terminating CPR efforts.

During CPR-ABC, prior to restoration of spontaneous circulation, some patients regain pupillary constriction and spontaneous respiratory movements, but almost never awareness. EEG activity during CPR cannot be monitored reliably, due to movement artifacts, and would be of poor prognosticating value, since it does not correlate with the degree and speed of neurologic recovery.

After restoration of spontaneous circulation, reactive pupils, increased responsiveness, spontaneous movements, and resumption of spontaneous breathing efforts are strong indications that there is some cerebral oxygenation. On the other hand, dilated, fixed pupils and absence of spontaneous breathing efforts for at least 1-2 hours, after the restoration of spontaneous circulation are usually, but not always, followed by brain death or recovery with severe brain damage. Dilated, fixed pupils, however, can also occur in the absence of cerebral death, as the result of brain contusion, skull fracture, intracranial hemorrhage, catecholamines given for resuscitation, or overdose with a hypnotic.

When the picture of brain death persists after restoration of spontaneous circulation, it is frequently associated with pressor resistant hypotension and cardiac arrest, secondary to medullary herniation from cerebral edema. If circulation continues, however, with or without vasopressors, brain death should not be certified until life support has been optimized and the patient's condition stabilized for at least 24 hours. Most patients who develop the criteria of brain death do so on the second post-arrest day, after varying degrees of initial neurologic improvement.

As a rough guide it is possible to say that most patients who begin to wake up within about 10 minutes after restoration of spontaneous circulation will recover with normal brain function. On the other hand, among those who show no purposeful response to painful stimuli (e.g., forceful pressure on the angles of the mandible), with no oculocephalic (doll's eye) reflex or oculovestibular (caloric) reflex by 6-12 hours after restoration of circulation, and who receive standard post-resuscitative care, the majority will suffer variable degrees of permanent brain damage (Bates). Such damage may range from minor psychologic-behavioral changes to the persistent vegetative state. It should be noted that the above mentioned tests of function may not be feasible under conditions where the use of anesthetics, other central nervous system depressants or relaxants are required for stabilization of the patient.

Even after recovery from anesthetics or relaxants, a persistent vegetative state (with active EEG and reflexes) cannot be diagnosed with certainty until 1-2 weeks of unconsciousness have elapsed after the CPR effort. This is particularly true when treatment has included new brain resuscitation methods, for use of these newer techniques has occasionally been followed by complete recovery, even in cases where there was 10-20 minutes of circulatory arrest in normothermia (or up to 40 minutes in hypothermia) and 1-2 weeks of unresponsiveness following CPR.

In *summary,* in potentially salvageable patients, termination of emergency resuscitation efforts is justified when there is solid evidence of irreversible cardiac arrest. It is not, however, justified solely on the basis of neurologic signs suggesting cerebral or brain death, since these signs are not reliable prognostic indicators during and immediately after CPR.

When to Terminate Long-Term Resuscitation (Table IX)

Triage in the context of resuscitation refers to the process of sorting critically ill patients in terms of expected outcome and possible treatment regimens. At Pittsburgh's Presbyterian-University Hospital, critical care triage is facilitated as follows: At least 2 physicians classify and periodically reclassify each ICU patient into 1 of 4 categories (Table IX) (Grenvik): (1) Total support (all ICU patients fall into this category at the time of ICU admission); (2) Full support short of CPR; (3) «letting die» (extra-ordinary measures withdrawn); and (4) brain death certification (all measures withdrawn). (Copy Table IX for your use).

How to Terminate Long-Term Resuscitation in Total Brain Death (Table X)

Brain death is the permanent loss of all integrated neuronal function, including cerebrum, brain stem, pons, mid-brain and cerebellum (Beecher). Brain death following cardiac arrest and CPR is usually the result of cerebral edema and consequent brain herniation, sometimes occurring after a brief period of neurologic improvement. Brain death is more likely to ensue after severe, prolonged insults or inadequate resuscitation. Destruction of the medullary centers results in intractable

TABLE IX

Recommended Critical Care Triage

Adapted from Grenvik, et al., 1978

1. Total support: For critically ill or injured patients in whom survival without persistent severe brain failure is expected. Vital organ systems, although usually affected, are not irreversibly damaged. Everything possible is done to reduce mortality and morbidity.

2. All but CPR: For patients with continuing brain function or hope for brain recovery, who have irreversible cardiopulmonary or other multiple organ failure, or are in the terminal stages of incurable diseases, e.g., advanced carcinomatosis. Everything possible is done for comfort. Prolongation of life is not carried beyond cardiac arrest. When this occurs, CPR is not provided and the patient is permitted to die.

3. No extraordinary measures, letting die: For patients where some forms of treatment seem meaningless, serving only to prolong death rather than life. Examples are patients with minimal brain function in whom there is no hope for improvement and thus no prospect for future human mentation. Extraordinary measures are not initiated for such patients or are discontinued if such discontinuation is not expected to result in immediate demise. Such extraordinary measures may include admission to the ICU; CPR; dysrhythmia control; tracheal intubation; mechanical ventilation; use of artificial organs; transplantation; blood transfusion; invasive monitoring; IV infusion of potent vasoactive drugs; and total parenteral nutrition. In some circumstances, the responsible physician may consider it medically sound and ethical to also withdraw gastric tube feeding, IV fluids and antibiotics. The conscious moribund hopeless patient is made comfortable and pain free.

4. Brain death determination and certification; termination of all life support: For patients with irreversible cessation of all brain function. Once brain death has been demonstrated by established criteria, the patient is declared dead and all therapy is stopped. If organ donation is being considered, cardiopulmonary support is continued until the required organs have been removed.

arterial hypotension and secondary cardiac arrest, in spite of use of vasopressors and artificial ventilation. Cardiac arrest usually occurs within 72 hours after the onset of the clinical picture of brain death, although in rare instances, hearts of artificially ventilated patients with brain death have been kept beating for up to one month. Nonetheless, once at least 2 licensed physicians have determined and certified total brain death, most ethical and legal views permit cessation of all treatment, including artificial ventilation (Mayrhofer, Beecher, Grenvik, Milhaud).

Specific criteria for determining brain death have been proposed by many groups. Such criteria should be established at the community, state or national level, but consistent with internationally accepted guidelines and practices. While there is agreement on concepts, guidelines differ concerning which tests are required. All require detailed neurologic examination. Different states' criteria may or may not demand repeat evaluation after 2,3,6 or 12 hours. Although most guidelines require EEG determination, in hospitals where reliable EEG tracings cannot be obtained, it is acceptable to determine brain death without proof of EEG silence, provided all other criteria are present. EEG tracings without artifacts are often impossible to obtain in ICUs.

Brain death criteria in use at the University of Pittsburgh since 1968 (Grenvik) are listed in Table X*. They include: Complete absence of cerebral and brain stem activity on two clinical examinations, performed at least two hours apart, in the absence of CNS depressants, relaxants or hypothermia. One isoelectric EEG recording, with and without auditory stimulation for at least 30 minutes, part of which must be with an amplification of 2 microvolts per mm. The EEG is usually obtained during the interval between the first and second clinical examination. Succinylcholine may be used to abolish muscle artifacts which interfere with the EEG tracing, but its effect must be absent (tested by nerve-muscle stimulator) before the subsequent clinical examination. There should be no spontaneous breathing activity within 3 minutes of apnea, with arterial PCO_2 permitted to rise to 50 mm Hg. Oxygen 100% should be given to prevent hypoxemia during the test, and blood gas analysis should be used for confirmation. Cranial nerve reflexes and responses, including pupillary reflexes, must be absent. The heart rate must not increase following atropine.

In short, all evidence of brain stem activity must be absent. Spinal cord activity (e.g., reflex spasms) however, may be present, as spinal cord neurons may remain viable after brain death. Two physicians must sign the certification document (Table X).

These criteria are only guidelines. Where EEG or blood gas monitoring is not available, carotid angiography and demonstration of the absence of intracranial perfusion is an acceptable alternative way to prove brain death. Where no laboratory determinations are available,

*See also ref. Amer. EEG Society, and Royal Colleges of U.K. (Bibliography).

clinical signs alone should suffice.

Brain death determination and certification should be done after stabilization of the patient in the ICU and after sufficient time has been allowed for the course of CNS deterioration to be assessed in an orderly fashion. Family consent is not required for certification of brain death.

Procedures to be fulfilled, once total brain death has been certified, will depend on local, regional and national criteria. In the U.S.A., once brain death has been certified, organs may be removed for transplantation, with signed consent from the family. All life support efforts including artificial ventilation are then discontinued and circulatory arrest is permitted to occur. (Copy Table X for your use).

TABLE X

Recommended Criteria for Brain Death Determination
Grenvik, et al., 1968, 1978

Note: The patient must be observed in the hospital during treatment of potentially correctable abnormalities (e.g. hypovolemic shock). Two clinical examinations must then be performed; the second no sooner than two hours after the first.

Date and time of 1st exam _____ 2nd exam_____

A. Coma of established cause and absence of induced hypothermia and central nervous system depressant drugs. A blood ethanol level and/or other appropriate toxicology studies should be performed if indicated. Body temperature should be recorded.

	1st exam	2nd exam
1. Body temperature	_____	_____
2. Blood ethanol	_____	_____
3. Toxicology studies	_____	_____

B. No spontaneous muscular movements and no evidence of decerebrate or decorticate posturing or shivering (in the absence of muscle relaxant). Spinal reflexes (stimuli causing movements) may be present.

TABLE X (continued)

C. Cranial Nerve Reflexes and Responses: 1st exam   2nd exam
   1. Pupils light-fixed   _____   _____
   2. Absent corneal reflexes   _____   _____
   3. Unresponsiveness to intensely painful
   stimuli, e.g. supraobital pressure   _____   _____
   4. Absent response to upper and lower
   airway stimulation (e.g. pharyngeal
   and endotracheal suctioning)   _____   _____
   5. Absent ocular response to head turning
   (no eye movement)   _____   _____
   6. Absent ocular response to irrigation
   of the ears with 50 ml of ice
   water (no eye movement)   _____   _____
D. Absence of spontaneous breathing movements for 3 minutes
   and $PaCO_2$ above 50 torr at end of test (in absence of muscle
   relaxant). If a history suggestive of dependence on a hypoxic
   stimulus for ventilation (e.g. emphysema) is present, the PaO_2 at
   end of test must be less than 50 torr.
   1. $PaCO_2$ at end of apnea test   _____   _____
   2. PaO_2 at end of apnea test   _____   _____
E. An isoelectric electroencephalogram
   recorded in part at full gain (see text).   _____   _____
F. Failure to increase heart rate by more than five per minute
   following 1 mg atropine intravenously:
   1. Heart rate before atropine   _____   _____
   2. Heart rate after atropine   _____   _____

C. Comments:_____

Certification
Having considered the above findings, we hereby certify the death of:

_____

Date _____ Time _____

     Physician's Signature   Names Printed

_____ Dr._____

_____ Dr._____

(This document should be signed by two physicians)

How to Terminate Long-Term Resuscitation in Vegetative State

(Table IX)

«Letting die» should be carried out according to medical, legal and ethical customs of the community. These determine the degree of care appropriate in hopeless, moribund patients.

The socio-economic tragedy of severely brain-damaged survivors is obvious, for such cases may impose an unbearable financial and emotional burden on the family. The decision to discontinue extraordinary means of life support is a medical one. It should be made by an experienced physician, who is thoroughly familiar with the entire case, in consultation with experienced specialists (e.g., anesthesiologist, critical care physician, neurologist), and should consider the patient's previously expressed wishes, the family's attitude, and the quality of life expected at best. Although one should not ask relatives to make the decision to let the patient die, their agreement with the physician's decision should be sought.

The criteria for brain death certification are objective and reliable. On the other hand, proof with 100% reliability in a given patient, of the persistent vegetative state (apallic syndrome), permanent severe neurologic deficit with consciousness, or irreversible coma without brain death, is usually not possible with presently available methods. Thus, the hopelessness of the situation must often be determined by a combination of published predictive criteria (none of which are 100% reliable) and clinical judgment.

While brain death certification calls for withdrawal of *all* life support measures, «letting die» (passive euthanasia, *not* active euthanasia) calls for discontinuance of *extraordinary measures* only (Table IX). Extraordinary measures may be defined differently in different countries, depending on priorities and available resources, which are finite everywhere. In most industrialized countries, extraordinary measures include mechanical ventilation, blood administration, dysrhythmia control, and life-supporting drugs, but may not include IV fluids, alimentation and airway control. In irreversible vegetative state antibiotics may justifiably be withheld as well.

The most common indications for «letting die» are irreversible coma due to cerebral (cortical) death (EEG silence without apnea); and persistent vegetative state (apallic syndrome). The latter differs from brain death in many ways, since the patient has an active EEG, cranial nerve reflexes and spontaneous breathing. He is simply «disconnected» from his surroundings.

Conclusion. The brain is the target organ of resuscitation. If resuscitation, through focusing on the brain, can reach beyond technologic advances and concern itself also with the quality of life, and other philosophic issues, it *can* be a positive force in the evolution of man.

Chapter IV

SPECIAL CONSIDERATIONS

Resuscitation of Infants and Children (Fig. 42)

For purposes of resuscitation, an infant is defined as under one year of age and a child as being one to eight years old. Children over eight years old may be treated with the techniques described for adult resuscitation. In terms of teaching and organization, it is worthwhile to coordinate teaching of neonatal and pediatric resuscitation with that of adult resuscitation. Trainees should learn adult resuscitation techniques before embarking on training programs for resuscitation for infants and children.

The sequence of steps of CPR and general resuscitation principles are the same for infants, children and adults. However, priorities and techniques differ somewhat when dealing with these different age groups, because of variations in size and cause of the emergency.

Cardiac arrest in children and infants is usually the result of asphyxia (e.g., suffocation by foreign body; near-drowning; trauma; burns; poisoning; upper airway infection; sudden infant death syndrome). Primary ventricular fibrillation or asystole is rare and, in newborn babies, almost unheard of. Thus, prevention of accidents is the most important principle of resuscitation in this age group. Once an emergency occurs, however, steps A and B of CPR are most important to prevent full-blown cardiac arrest.

Basic Life Support Without Equipment

If the child is unconscious, proceed with the same sequence of steps as in adults. Use head-tilt, by neck-lift or by chin-support, whichever works better (Fig. 41). Do not use extreme backward-tilt of the head, as this can narrow the infant's upper air passage. Often simple head-tilt is all that is needed to open the airway. If not, add gentle jaw thrust. Do not close the infant's mouth.

Resuscitation of Infants and Children
Steps A and B, Without Equipment

1 Open the *airway*. (Head-tilt or neck-lift. Do not hyperextend the infant's neck.)
2 If the infant is not *breathing*, begin artificial ventilation.
  a Encircle the infant's *mouth and nose* with your mouth.
  b Use *small, gentle* inflations at a rapid rate. (It is easy to rupture an infant's lungs, so use only puffs from your cheeks.)
  c Watch to determine if the chest rises.
  d Take your mouth off the infant's face between inflations, to avoid overinflating his lungs.

Rate of inflation
Infants: 1 every 2 seconds (30 per minute)
Children: 1 every 3 seconds (20 per minute)

Although air is easily blown into the infant's stomach, nonetheless do *not* maintain manual pressure on the epigastrium, as this can provoke regurgitation. Press over the epigastrium for gastric decompressions only if abdominal distention makes ventilation impossible (and then do it only after the child has been turned on his side); accompany pressure over the epigastrium with gentle clearing of the pharynx by finger or suction.

Resuscitation of Infants and Children
Step C, Without Equipment

1 Steps A and B initiated, with four lung inflations, –
2 Feel for a *pulse.* (In a child, check the carotid artery. In an infant, check the brachial or femoral artery. Precordial pulses are unreliable.)
3 If there is no pulse, start *external cardiac compressions.*
  a *Site:* In the infant compress the *midsternum (*an infant's heart lies higher in the chest); for the child, press slightly below the midsternum, but higher than one would for an adult.
  b *Method:* In the infant use 2-3 fingers placed on the midsternum (between the nipples) and compress 1.5 — 2.5 cm; in the child, use the heel of one hand to compress the sternum 2.5 — 3.0 cm.
  c *Rate of sternal compressions:*
    In the infant compress 100 times per minute
    In the child compress 80 times per minute
  d *Rate of ventilations to compressions:* 1:5.

Step F, Defibrillation

1 Use external defibrillator chest electrodes (with built-in EKG electrodes) of 4.5 cm diameter for infants, and 8 cm diameter for children.
2 Treat ventricular fibrillation (and ventricular tachycardia with unconsciousness) by external countershock with 2 joules/kg.
3 If above fails, repeat shock with 4 joules/kg. Before increasing the dose further, improve oxygenation, give epinephrine and correct arterial pH.

In the case of acute airway obstruction, when there has been a history of fever and barking cough, one should suspect *croup or epiglottitis.* The usual measures for managing foreign body obstruction are contra-indicated in such cases, and the patient should instead be rushed to the hospital, where emergency tracheal intubation or tracheotomy may be required. Oxygen should be given en route, if available. Pre-hospital

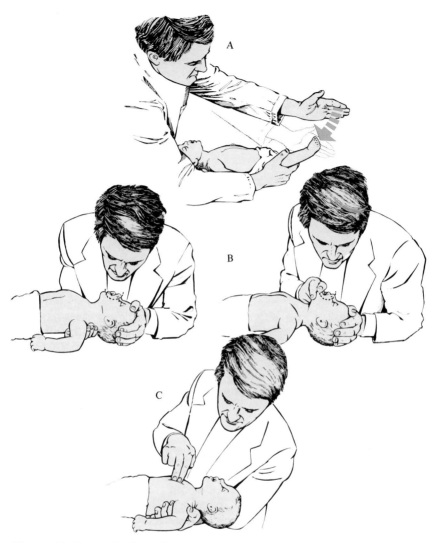

Figure 42: Resuscitation of the newborn

(A) Stimulate sole of foot for arousal.

(B) If the baby's breathing is inadequate and bag-mask-oxygen unit is not available, perform mouth-to-mouth-nose ventilation with head-tilt by neck-lift (left) or head-tilt by chin support (right). Ventilate with puffs from your cheeks.

(C) If no pulse can be palpated in the brachial or femoral artery, or if the heart rate is below 100 per minute, give external cardiac compressions with two fingers over the infant's midsternum at a rate of *about 100 per minute. Interpose one lung inflation after every fifth sternal compression, for one or two operators. Support chest with one hand to maintain head-tilt during Steps B and C; this may make it unnecessary to switch one hand to forehead during ventilations. An alternate method (not shown) for chest compressions is to encircle the chest with both hands, with the fingers at the back and thumbs pressing over the sternum.*

attempts at tracheal intubation in such cases should be by an experienced operator and as a last step.

When circumstances suggest that obstruction has been caused by a *foreign body,* and the child is conscious, he should be encouraged to cough up the foreign body. If cough is ineffective, or if the child becomes cyanotic or unconscious, a combination of gentle finger sweeps of the pharynx, back blows and chest thrusts should be used. Abdominal thrusts are *not* recommended in infants and children, because of the danger of causing internal injuries. For back blows, the infant is placed over the rescuer's arm with the head lowered; the child is placed over the kneeling rescuer's thighs with the head lowered. Chest thrusts are applied like external cardiac compressions with the patient supine. If possible, the finger sweep should be carried out under direct vision, with one hand performing tongue-jaw-lift, and the other clearing the pharynx (Fig. 6). Blind finger probing may further impact the foreign body. After carrying out these procedures to remove the foreign body, try again to inflate the lungs with mouth-to-mouth-and-nose, and repeat the sequence as described for adults (pg. 26).

Resuscitation of Newborns

When cardiac arrest in the newborn occurs outside the hospital, in the absence of health care personnel, the basic life support measures summarized above are the only ones available for treating newborn infants in distress. Wherever possible, deliveries should be conducted in hospital with safe obstetric and newborn resuscitation services. If conducted outside hospital, at least the presence of personnel experienced in newborn resuscitation techniques, including the use of equipment, is essential.

The importance of neonatal resuscitation is evident from the fact that any degree of asphyxia in the first few minutes of life can cripple a child for life. Airway obstruction by mucus, blood, meconium or the tongue; brain damage during traumatic birth; drugs given to the mother; and blood loss from cord compression or hemorrhage — all can result in asphyxia and shock in the newborn infant, and lasting brain damage.

Evaluation of the neonate with *Apgar's scoring system* has been adopted worldwide and is recommended as a simple, uniform way of assessing the infant's condition. This is best done at one and five minutes after full delivery. However, *resuscitation should never wait for determination of the Apgar score.* The scoring system uses five objective signs which are evaluated and scored with 0, 1 or 2 — making the best score 10, and the worst score 0 (Table XI).

TABLE XI

Apgar Scoring System

For evaluating Newborn Infant
(e.g., at 1 and 5 minutes after full delivery)

Clinical Sign	Score		
	0 points	1 point	2 points
A: Appearance (Color)	blue, pale	body pink, extremities blue	completely pink
P: Pulse	absent	less than 100	over 100
G: Grimace (reflex irritability)	no response	grimaces	cries
A: Activity (muscle tone)	limp	some flexion of extremities	active motion
R: Respiratory effort	absent	slow, irregular	good, strong cry
Total Score	worst: 0		best: 10

Score 10 — optimal condition
Score 6 or less — depression; resuscitative measures required

Normal *deliveries,* and particularly complicated deliveries, should be managed in a way that permits immediate treatment in the event of asphyxia, hypothermia, shock, acidemia and hypoglycemia (Abouleish).

Immediately after delivery of the infant's head, gently clear the nose and pharynx with suction. Use a hand operated bulb aspirator or an alternative mechanical device, ensuring that the vacuum does not exceed 30 cm H_2O. The catheter used for suction may also be used to check for nasal-choanal patency.

If the infant is breathing and pink upon full delivery, quickly dry his skin and place him on his side, with the head tilted backward, against the mother's body to prevent heat loss. If he needs resuscitation, keep the baby supine (horizontal, face-up) with his head held in moderate backward tilt. Add jaw thrust or a pharyngeal tube if necessary. If his breathing is shallow or cyanosis is present, use exhaled air ventilation; this may require skillfully adjusted assisted breathing superimposed on the patients own respirations (when the patient breathes in, you breathe out). Cyanosis as a sign of hypoxemia is more reliable in infants than in adults, because of the infants higher hemoglobin content.

For neonatal *respiratory resuscitation* in the hospital, a bag-mask-oxygen unit is recommended — using either a valveless to-and-fro unit (which requires an anesthesiologist's skills) or the infant version of a self-refilling bag-valve-mask unit with oxygen reservoir (e.g., Laerdal infant unit). The bag-mask unit should have a pressure limiting pop-off valve, preset at 30-35 cm H_2O, with a 60 cm H_2O override, since high pressure may be necessary for initial lung inflation. In the absen.e of a pop-off valve, an airway pressure gauge should be attached to the bag-valve-mask unit and observed carefully in order to avoid pressures over 30 cm H_2O. The unit should have a low dead space, an effectively sealing infant mask, and an oxygen reservoir permitting delivery of 50-100% oxygen to the infant. Manually triggered oxygen-powered ventilation devices are not recommended.

When ventilation by mask fails, intubate the trachea, preferably using a tapered Cole endotracheal tube size 12-14 French, Tbl. II. Initiate mouth-to-tracheal tube ventilation. Oxygen enrichment of your exhaled air can be accomplished by filling your own mouth with oxygen via a nasal or oral cannula.

If the baby is stained by meconium during delivery, first clear the pharynx by suction, immediately as the head is delivered, prior to his starting to breathe. If you are subsequently in doubt about the baby's oxygenation, intubate the trachea and, with your mouth, apply suction directly to the tracheal tube (via a suction trap if available), while withdrawing the tube. Re-intubate, inflate the lungs with puffs via the tube, and repeat suction and lung inflations until ventilation and oxygenation appear adequate.

Endotracheal *intubation* and ventilation with oxygen by mouth-to-tube or bag-valve-tube are indicated if, in spite of assisted ventilation by bag-mask-oxygen, oronasal suctioning, warming and external stimuli, breathing remains depressed or the heart rate drops below 100 per minute.

Prolonged respiratory distress calls for continuous positive pressure breathing, which is increasingly also recommended as a prophylactic measure in severely premature or asphyxiated infants, to prevent the development of respiratory distress syndrome. Spontaneous breathing with positive airway pressure is possible via mask or nasal prongues, while IPPV with PEEP requires a tracheal tube. Both are specialized measures to be carried out wherever possible in neonatal intensive care units (Chapter 1B) (Gregory).

If respiratory resuscitation fails to restore adequate circulation, external cardiac compressions for assisted circulation should be considered, whenever the heart rate is below 100 per minute. In circulatory distress, a catheter should be inserted into the umbilical artery for drug and fluid administration, blood gas monitoring, and pressure monitoring. Insert a 3.5-5 French catheter into the umbilical stump, via one of its two thick-walled arteries, 2-3 cm beyond the point where blood returns freely (Kitterman).

If there is *hypotension,* as measured by umbilical artery transducer or infant-cuff technique, in spite of adequate oxygenation, infuse a 15 ml/kg dose of 5% albumin, lactated Ringer's solution or blood. In addition give dextrose 10-25% in water (an initial dose of 0.5 gm/kg), since hypoglycemia is common in neonates. Fluid overload must be avoided, as there is little room for error in treating the neonate. Take steps to restore the body temperature to normal.

Determine arterial pH, PCO_2 and hemoglobin and calculate base deficit. Correct the latter *slowly* with sodium bicarbonate, in milliequivalent doses equal to base deficit in milliequivalents per liter times 25 % of body weight in kg. Rapid bicarbonate administration can lead to cerebral acidosis from increased CO_2 and to intracranial hemorrhage from hypernatremia.

If there is cardiac arrest, severe asphyxia or shock, and blood gas analyses are not available, *slowly* inject sodium bicarbonate 1-2 mEq/kg diluted 1:1 with 10% dextrose in water into the umbilical artery. For shock add intravenous 10% dextrose in Ringer's solution. Bicarbonate 1 mEq/kg may be repeated every 10 minutes of arrest. In cardiac arrest, epinephrine is also indicated in 1:10,000 dilution (1 mg/10 ml), 0.1 ml/kg intravenously.

Cardiac resuscitation is not always justified in clinically dead newborn infants. Obviously, where there is only transient pulselessness following a complicated delivery, a brief period of closed-chest CPR may quickly restart the asphyxiated asystolic heart and therefore is justified. After CPR for prolonged pulselessness, however, irreversible brain damage (cerebral palsy) is almost certain to follow, since cardiac arrest in the newborn infant occurs secondary to asphyxia or shock, which are usually associated with prolonged traumatic labor. Obviously, in infants and children beyond the first few hours of life (provided there are no defects incompatible with ultimate survival) sudden pulselessness should be treated with all-out CPR.

In the newborn, respiratory resuscitation, fluid and acid-base control, temperature control and treatment of hypoglycemia must be carried out vigorously; but prolonged cardiac resuscitation efforts are unwise as they may result in the survival of a severely brain-damaged child.

Drugs for resuscitation of *infants and children* are the same as those used for adults, but the dosages are slightly different.

Drug Dosages for Resuscitation of Neonates, Infants and Children

Drug	Dose
Epinephrine (adrenaline)	0.1 ml/kg of a 1:10,000 dilution IV
Sodium bicarbonate	1 mEq/kg IV
Calcium chloride 10 %	1 ml/5 kg IV
Lidocaine (Xylocaine, lignocaine)	0.5 mg/kg IV, or as titrated infusion
Norepinephrine (Levophed)	Titrated infusion — 1 mg/500 ml — infants 2 mg/500 ml — children
Metaraminol (Aramine)	Titrated infusion: 25 mg/500 ml
Isoproterenol (Isuprel)	Titrated infusion: 1-5 mg/500 ml
Atropine	0.03 mg/kg IV
Naloxone (Narcan)	0.01 mg/kg IV

Respiratory stimulants (coramine, cardiazol, picrotoxin, etc.) are not indicated in neonatal resuscitation!

Equipment available in the *delivery room* should include adjustable suction with vacuum manometer; suction catheters size 5, 6 and 8 French; bag-valve-mask unit with mask sizes 0 and 1 and with oxygen reservoir; oropharyngeal tubes sizes 0, 00 and 000; Cole tracheal tubes 2.5-3.0 mm diameter (sizes 12 and 14 French) with stylet; laryngoscope with straight blades sizes 0 and 1; an oxygen source; an umbilical artery catheterization tray with catheters 2.5 and 5 French; three-way stopcocks; drugs; and intravenous fluids.

Monitoring, resuscitation and intensive care of the fetus and neonate in hospitals are highly specialized fields and therefore beyond the scope of this manual. We would like to stress, however, that resuscitation services for newborn infants should integrate basic life support, advanced life support and post-resuscitative intensive therapy as part of *community-wide* emergency medical services. All general advanced life support facilities should be staffed and equipped to provide basic and advanced life support, not only for adults but also for infants and children (Chapter VI). Although resuscitation attempts for infants and children are required less often than for adults, successful resuscitation of a child provides a better opportunity for restoring long-term survival with quality of life. Conversely, inadequate resuscitation of a child is more likely to result in lifelong brain-damaged survival.

It is recommended that all hospitals with obstetric services be equipped and staffed for advanced neonatal resuscitation and for transfer of the infant with life support to a neonatal intensive care unit. Ideally, neonatal intensive care services should be established on a regional basis, as should obstetric units for identified high-risk pregnancies.

Within hospitals with obstetric services, newborn resuscitation should be organized and quality controlled by an inter-disciplinary committee. For neonatal resuscitation at least two persons are required, one to ventilate and intubate and the other to monitor, insert catheters, medicate, and perform cardiac compressions if necessary.

Witnessed Sudden Cardiac Death (Fig. 43)

There are a number of special considerations and controversies that apply to the management of witnessed sudden cardiac arrest, among them: (1) Use of the C-A-B sequence in place of the usual A-B-C order; (2) Empirical electric countershock («blind defibrillation») in the absence of an EKG tracing; (3) Cough-CPR; and (4) Precordial thump. Of these four techniques, the present author endorses (3) and (4).

Cough-CPR

When sudden ventricular fibrillation without gasping or coughing induces cardiac arrest instantaneously, the victim becomes unconscious within 10-15 seconds. Spontaneous vigorous gasping or — even better — repetitive, vigorous coordinated coughing, can produce blood pressure fluctuations and small amounts of blood flow due to intrathoracic pressure fluctuations. The deep inhalation (Mueller maneuver) produces a thoracic diastole; the subsequent glottic closure and pressure buildup (Valsalva maneuver) produces a thoracic systole. In the cardiac catheterization laboratory, patients have been coached to stay conscious by coughing for up to 90 seconds of ventricular fibrillation, after which they were defibrillated (Criley). Cough-CPR is presently under investigation in animals and patients. It is not yet known how long following sudden onset ventricular fibrillation active coughing can maintain sufficient oxygen transport to the brain to keep the patient conscious.

This author recommends: (1) Health care personnel should be taught to encourage repetitive coughing when a monitored patient suddenly develops ventricular fibrillation; this should be considered an emergency standby measure until a defibrillator is available. (2) Selected patients at risk of sudden cardiac death could be taught, «if you feel like your heart has stopped, call for help and cough forcefully once every second, with deep breaths in between coughs; this might keep you conscious until help arrives». Although the efficacy of this recommendation has not yet been examined, cough-CPR is at present the only possible self-help measure available for sudden cardiac death. When considering trials of cough-CPR one must keep in mind potential harm from coughing in the absence of cardiac arrest, such as the possibility of inducing hypoxemia, bradycardia or ventricular fibrillation in patients with severe heart disease; and the possibility of syncope from a sustained Valsalva phase of cough.

Precordial Thump (Fig. 43)

There is no evidence that the electric current produced in the heart by precordial thump is strong enough to terminate ventricular fibrillation. There is on the other hand, some experimental and clinical evidence that one precordial thump can convert sudden ventricular tachycardia back to sinus rhythm (Pennington); the thump can also, however, unexpectedly induce ventricular fibrillation (Redding). In severe bradycardia or asystole from heart block (Adams-Stokes syndrome), repetitive precordial thumping, if started within about 30 seconds of syncope, can often induce spontaneous cardiac contractions. Standard external cardiac compressions, however, can accomplish the same, and in addition circulate blood, which thumps cannot do. In severe bradycardia, precordial thumping or external cardiac compressions do not have to be synchronized with spontaneous cardiac contractions. Repetitive thumping, also called «fist-pacing», is less painful than sternal compressions.

Precordial thumping can neither defibrillate nor stimulate cardiac contractions when the heart is anoxic; thus thumping is not a substitute for external cardiac compressions and adequate ventilation.

The recommended *sequence* of techniques is as follows:

In witnessed cardiac arrest *without* EKG monitoring, use standard CPR: head-tilt, ventilation, palpation for pulse, external cardiac compressions,etc. If he becomes unconscious and continues to breathe while you find the carotid pulse absent, go straight to step C (external cardiac compressions), since he is providing steps A and B himself. If he has a very slow heart rate (less than 40 per minute) or is known to have heart block, and develops syncope, use the less painful repetitive thumping (fist pacing) when he is conscious, and external cardiac compressions when he is unconscious. Apply repetitive thumping at a rate of about 60 per minute. Ask an assistant to give atropine or isoproterenol I.V. and initiate insertion of an intravenous pacemaker, once the diagnosis of heart block has been established.

In witnessed cardiac arrest *with* EKG monitoring, treat ventricular tachycardia or ventricular fibrillation with immediate electric countershock, without first starting CPR steps ABC. As soon as ventricular tachycardia or ventricular fibrillation is suspected, feel for the carotid or femoral pulse. If it is absent, apply one countershock. Immediately recheck the pulse. If he remains pulseless, tilt his head backward, give 4 quick lung inflations, check the pulse again, begin external cardiac compressions, and continue with standard CPR. Repeat the countershocks as needed (Chapter II).

If you see ventricular tachycardia on the EKG tracing and find the patient pulseless, and a defibrillator is not immediately available, apply one precordial thump. If this does not terminate ventricular tachycardia or ventricular fibrillation, continue CPR and use the defibrillator when it arrives.

If you see sudden severe bradycardia or asystole on the EKG tracing, give repetitive precordial thumps (at the rate of about 60 per minute) while the patient is conscious, and switch to standard CPR when he becomes unconscious.

In *unwitnessed* cardiac arrest and in witnessed arrest in infants and small children precordial thumping is *not* recommended.

In sudden witnessed cardiac arrest without EKG monitoring, but where a DC defibrillator is available, apply *empirically* one external electric *countershock* and continue with CPR. This situation has become rare, since most portable defibrillators include EKG monitors with EKG

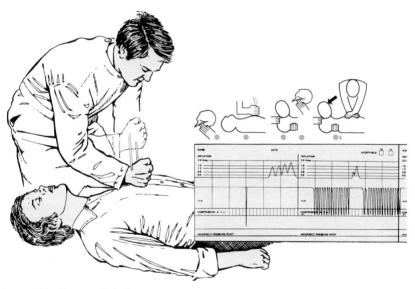

Figure 43: Precordial thump

From a height of 8-12 inches above the chest, deliver a sharp quick single blow over the midportion of the sternum, using the fleshy bottom portion of the fist.

Inset shows manikin tracing of demonstration of a thump as first measure in witnessed, EKG-monitored sudden cardiac arrest. Because this failed to restore a spontaneous pulse, CPR was continued as shown. For indications for precordial thump, see text.

electrodes incorporated in the defibrillating paddles.

Treatment of witnessed, monitored, sudden ventricular fibrillation or ventricular tachycardia by immediate external electric countershock without preliminary CPR steps ABC has become routine in cardiac units. This method is effective so long as the heart is oxygenated, i.e., for about 30 to 60 seconds after the onset of pulselessness. Therefore, each patient at risk of arrest, should have a defibrillator in immediate readiness.

Open-Chest Cardiopulmonary Resuscitation (Fig. 44)

Cardiac resuscitation via thoracotomy was practiced widely in hospitals before the introduction of closed-chest CPR in 1960, and the earlier technique produced high survival rates with good brain function (Boehm, Beck, Leighninger, Dripps, Stephenson). Direct cardiac compressions produce better blood flow than sternal compressions, since the latter increase overall intrathoracic pressure which in turn increases venous pressure simultaneously with arterial pressure. The open-chest technique produces higher arterio-venous perfusion pressures, and when cardiac massage is necessary for prolonged periods, also a better chance for sustaining cerebral viability and restoring spontaneous circulation (DelGuercio, McKenzie, Bircher, Alifimoff).

In addition, open-chest CPR permits direct palpation and observation of the heart, which helps guide drug and fluid therapy and electric countershock in difficult protracted CPR efforts. Finally, the open chest also permits direct compression of a bleeding site in intrathoracic exsanguination and, in cases of intra-abdominal hemorrhage, allows temporary compression or clamping of the thoracic aorta above the diaphragm.

For most cases of cardiac arrest, closed-chest CPR has replaced open-chest CPR, because the former can be started without delay, and can be performed by persons not trained in surgical techniques (i.e., outside the hospital). Many physicians fear the possible complications associated with thoracotomy, such as injury to heart and great vessels, and infection. In the hands of physicians with the necessary skills, equipment and facilities, however, the open-chest CPR approach is safe, and it is hemodynamically superior to the closed-chest technique.

Open-chest CPR is *indicated* (in the hands of trained physicians only) in circumstances for which it may be the only effective method of restoring life:

1 When you suspect intrathoracic pathology such as uncontrollable hemorrhage associated with cardiac arrest; particularly from penetrating wounds of the chest, crushing chest injury or following cardiothoracic surgery; and when you suspect cardiac tamponade.

2 When you cannot produce a palpable femoral or carotid pulse with sternal compressions, as occasionally is the case in patients with chest

or spine deformities or severe emphysema with barrel-chest.

3 As the last step in treating intractable ventricular fibrillation or electromechanical dissociation, when prolonged closed-chest CPR and repeated external defibrillation attempts have failed; this may be the case in suspected massive pulmonary thromboembolism (when the open technique permits breaking-up or removing the embolus) or in deep hypothermia (when the open technique permits direct rewarming of the heart for defibrillation).

4 For cardiac arrest in the operating room in a patient whose chest is already open (Stephenson).

Technique of Open-Chest CPR
(Intubated patients only)

1 *Cut* through skin and muscles directly overlying the fourth or fifth left intercostal space. Pierce the intercostal structures bluntly with a knife handle or bandage scissors and tear open the intercostal space with your fingers. Insert a rib spreader if available.

2 Immediately *compress the heart,* without at first opening the pericardium, by placing the fingers of the right hand behind the heart and the thenar and thumb in front of the heart. Take care not to pierce the atrium or ventricle with your thumb. If the heart is large, use one hand behind and one hand in front of the heart to compress it.

3 Usually one can diagnose ventricular fibrillation, inject drugs and defibrillate through a closed pericardium (one can see and feel the wormlike motions of ventricular fibrillation). Whenever you are not certain, however, and thus choose to open the pericardium, take care not to interrupt compressions or injure the heart or vagus nerve. In intractable ventricular fibrillation or when the first dose of epinephrine has failed to restart cardiac action, open the pericardium to allow direct inspection of the heart and to prevent injury to coronary vessels from multiple needle punctures.

4 *Drug Therapy*
a When drugs are necessary, they should be injected into the cavity of the left ventricle, *not* into the myocardium!
b Start with epinephrine, 0.5mg/70 kg.
c Atropine and lidocaine may also be given safely via the intracardiac route.
d Do *not* give bicarbonate intracardiac — use the intravenous route.

5 *Defibrillation*
a Use two *insulated paddle electrodes* (about five inch diameter for adults, with saline-soaked pad attached to each paddle).
b Place one electrode behind the left ventricle, the other over the

anterior surface of the heart.

c *DC countershock* is preferred. The operator should have control over the switch that releases the countershock.

d Start with 0.5 watt-seconds (joules)/kg body weight *(25-50 watt-seconds* in the average adult). If shock is ineffective at this low energy level, increase the energy level gradually with subsequent shocks. High energy shocks applied directly to the heart are more likely than external countershock to produce heat damage, including myocardial burns.

Note: Alternating current (AC) countershocks applied directly to the heart, although obsolete, are also effective. They should deliver 110 to 220 volt shocks of 0.1 to 0.25 seconds' duration. This can be improvised, in the absence of a defibrillator, by connecting 2 metal spoons — held in rubber-gloved hands — to a cord with regular male wall plugs, and then have a helper briefly plug the cord into a wall outlet.

In suspected *cardiac tamponade,* if time permits and the patient is not yet pulseless, rapid drainage of the pericardiac sac by needle puncture (alongside the xiphoid) may obviate the need for thoracotomy. If the diagnosis is uncertain, the chest and pericardium should be opened and direct cardiac compressions started.

Open-chest cardiac resuscitation should not be undertaken without endotracheal controlled ventilation with IPPV and PEEP, by a physician who is familiar with the pathophysiology of the open thorax and knowledgeable about thoracotomy.

Cardiac Arrest due to Exsanguination

Exsanguination usually leads to an agonal state (no pulse, gasping) and, after loss of more than 50% of blood volume, to clinical death in asystole (Negovsky). Resuscitative efforts may subsequently elicit ventricular fibrillation.

Resuscitation consists of the *simultaneous* application of the following (Kirimli, Torpey, Negovski):

1 *Ventilation* (with oxygen if available) plus external cardiac compressions.

2 *Control of hemorrhage* — by external compression of the bleeding site; tourniquet; shock trousers (MAST suit, see Chapter IC); laparotomy; or thoracotomy.

3 *Massive intravenous infusion,* through large-bore catheters or needles, of the most immediately available plasma substitute — sodium chloride, lactated Ringer's solution, dextran, hydroxyethyl starch or albumin. Infuse electrolyte solution in quantities up to 4 times the blood volume lost, or colloid solution in quantities up to a volume equal to estimated loss, until spontaneous cardiac action has restarted.

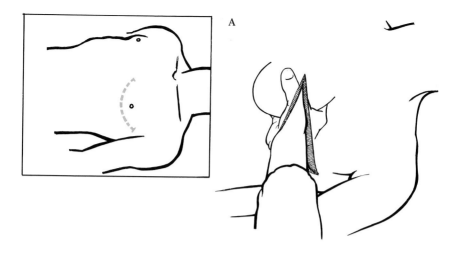

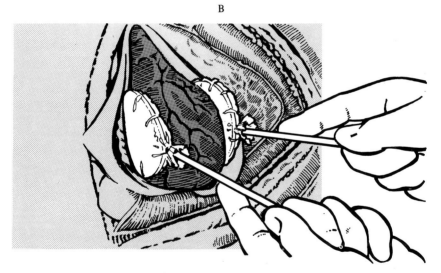

Figure 44: Open-chest cardiopulmonary resuscitation

(A) Open the chest at the fourth or fifth left intercostal space (inset).
Grasp and rhythmically compress the heart as described in the text (from
Johnson, Surgery of the Chest, Chicago, Year Book Medical Publ., 1952).

(B) Internal direct electric defibrillation. When fibrillation is felt, apply
the electrodes and countershock, first with the pericardium closed. (If
possible, have electrodes prepared with tied-on saline-soaked gauze).
Apply the internal electrodes as illustrated, wearing rubber gloves, and
release the shock (see text).

Then reduce the flow rate. Banked blood or packed red cells (group 0, rhesus negative; or typed and cross-matched) are optional. If used, blood should preferably be given via a blood warmer and micropore filter. Immediate massive infusion of plasma substitutes is more effective than delayed infusion of blood!

4 *Epinephrine* (1 mg) and *sodium bicarbonate* (1 mEq/kg) should be administered into the running I.V. without mixing (3, above).

5 *EKG monitoring* and defibrillation as indicated.

In experimental animals with asystole from exsanguination, spontaneous cardiac activity is usually restored during external cardiac compressions when about 50% of shed blood volume has been replaced. The other 50%, plus an addditional 10-20% of estimated blood volume to compensate for vasodilation and capillary leakage, should be restored more slowly, while monitoring arterial pressure, central venous pressure (and pulmonary artery pressure,optional), and blood gases if possible, to avoid overloading. When exsanguination arrest is reversed with electrolyte solutions only, colloid must be added within 1-2 hours, since salt solutions do not remain in the intravascular compartment (Takaori).

Hemoglobin is usually not needed to restart the circulation, provided that the hemorrhage is controlled. Rapid exsanguination leaves 40 to 50% of total red cell mass in the body. Continued blood loss, accompanied by further wash-out of hemoglobin with plasma substitutes, however, may reduce hematocrit below 20%. If this is the case, typed and cross-matched blood, if immediately available, should be used in conjunction with plasma substitutes. After restoration of spontaneous circulation and control of hemorrhage, a hematocrit of 25-35 % should be restored and clotting factors replaced as needed.

Intra-abdominal hemorrhage should be treated, to prevent cardiac arrest, with application of a pressure suit (MAST suit) (Kaplan). The suit should stay inflated at 100 mmHg until the team is ready for laparotomy and massive infusion. In case of cardiac arrest, left thoracotomy and clamping of the lower thoracic aorta can stop the hemorrhage before deflation of the pressure suit (Stewart).

In experimental conditions with use of warm oxygenated, heparinized blood with epinephrine (Negovsky), exsanguination cardiac arrest can be reversed somewhat more rapidly and with less volume by using the *intra-arterial* route of infusion. This can restart the heart even without cardiac compressions, due to retrograde perfusion of the coronary arteries. These conditions do not apply in the clinical setting. When clinically available plasma substitutes or cold banked blood was used via the arterial route in animals, the heart did not restart without cardiac compressions. On the other hand, massive venous infusion of plasma substitutes at room temperature plus CPR are effective in restarting the heart, as the infused fluids are oxygenated and diluted in passage through the lungs (Kirimli). Intraarterial infusion also carries with it the hazards of delay due to arterial cutdown; retrograde cerebral air or thromboembolism, even with use of a peripheral artery; and loss of limb from arterial thrombosis. However, when a large artery is readily available, as in a large open wound during a surgical operation, a trial of arterial pressure infusion during compressions may be justified.

Near-Drowning

Victims of near-drowning may or may not have water in their lungs, depending upon whether reflex laryngospasm prevented aspiration. In any case, however, reoxygenation should *not* be delayed by attempts to drain fluid from the lungs. A good swimmer can start mouth-to-mouth or mouth-to-nose resuscitation while treading water; otherwise start mouth-to-mouth ventilation while standing in shallow water, placing the victim's head and chest over your knee. Sternal compressions are not possible until the victim is removed from the water.

If neck injury is suspected following diving into the shallow water, try to float the victim onto a backboard before removing him from the water. If mouth-to-mouth ventilation is needed, use jaw thrust with moderate backward tilt of the head, asking a helper to hold head-neck-chest aligned, to avoid aggravating a spinal cord injury. Do not flex the neck.

Swimming rescue should only be attempted by strong swimmers. Others should quickly find a floating device. Teaching rapid rescue from water is as important as teaching resuscitation.

In general, the principles of CPR should be followed as previously outlined. Clear the pharynx. Water and vomitus may drain by gravity before and during resuscitative efforts. If after the victim has been removed from the water his abdomen is distended, turn him briefly on his side and compress the upper abdomen to expel water and gas; or turn him to the prone position, lifting him, with your hands under his stomach, to force water out («breaking» the victim). These efforts should not be routine, as they may delay reoxygenation and, if performed, should be rapid. Switch ventilation from exhaled air to 100 per cent oxygen as soon as possible, as pulmonary changes occur with even small amounts of inhaled water.

Inhalation of fresh water causes hemodilution and pulmonary shunting from surfactant failure; inhalation of sea water causes leakage of plasma into the alveoli (i.e., pulmonary edema). Both require sophisticated prolonged respiratory care with IPPV plus optimized PEEP, using first 100% O_2 and later oxygen concentrations to achieve an arterial PO_2 of at least 100 mm Hg. Even when cardiac arrest develops during submersion, resuscitation is possible (Redding).

Hospital admission is mandatory, even if the victim recovers consciousness at the scene or during transportation. Late pulmonary edema is not unusual, and there may be a variety of changes in blood electrolytes depending on the composition of the fluid inhaled.

While the pulmonary lesion of near-drowning is now reversible with advanced respiratory intensive care and other life support measures, the post-ischemic-anoxic brain damage remains a limiting factor. Thus, brain resuscitation (Chapter III) is important in patients who do not begin to wake up within a few minutes of restoration of spontaneous circulation. Usually these are victims with healthy hearts, and barbiturate therapy and therapeutic moderate hypothermia are less hazardous than in cardiac patients. Do not give up resuscitative efforts easily, since recovery from near-drowning with complete restoration of central nervous system function has been reported even after prolonged periods of submersion, particularly when there is hypothermia induced by drowning in cold water (Siebke). In such instances, rewarming should be gradual. Blood electrolyte changes are evanescent and no obstacle to resuscitation (Modell). Severe mixed acidemia calls for controlled hyperventilation and titrated sodium bicarbonate I.V..

Myocardial Ischemia and Infarction. Sudden Cardiac Death

Coronary artery disease is the most frequent cause of «sudden cardiac death», which is defined as «unexpected cardiac arrest without symptoms or with symptoms of less than one hour's duration» (Cobb). Two-thirds of sudden cardiac deaths due to coronary ischemia occur outside of hospitals. Although three-fourths of these victims have advanced coronary artery disease at autopsy, in more than 50% myocardial infarction is not evident as a precipitating factor; these 50% suffer probably sudden ventricular fibrillation, triggered by temporary focal myocardial ischemia in «hearts too good to die» (Beck). Cases of sudden cardiac death with or without myocardial infarction (the latter usually being diagnosed after hospital admission) require CPR basic life support by bystanders, followed promptly by advanced life support from ambulance personnel attempting to restart spontaneous circulation at the scene (Lund; Cobb).

Sudden ventricular fibrillation is often preceded by unrecognized ventricular extrasystoles (premature ventricular complexes) (PVCs) or ventricular tachycardia. These tachydysrhythmias are sometimes triggered by bradycardia, particularly in acute myocardial infarction. Therefore in uncomplicated acute myocardial infarction, suspected or proven, the following measures are crucial for the prevention of sudden cardiac death (Amer. Heart Assoc., Cobb, Valentine).

Prevention of Sudden Cardiac Death
in Suspected Acute Myocardial Ischemia

1 Administer *oxygen* at the earliest possible moment to any adult with chest pain.

2 Establish a keep-open *I.V. line* with 5% dextrose in water.
3 Begin EKG *monitoring.*
4 *Treat pain*
    a 50% oxygen/50% nitrous oxide self-administered by patient.
    b if nitrous oxide unavailable and if the patient is not hypotensive, give morphine in small, titrated doses of 2-5 mg I.V. each.
5 *PVC prophylaxis* — lidocaine infusion 1-4 mg/70 kg per minute.
6 *Treat PVCs* with lidocaine bolus (75-100 mg/70 kg I.V.) if —
    a there are more than 6 PVCs per minute
    b there are multifocal PVCs
    c there are two or more PVCs in a row
    d PVCs fall on a T wave (R-on-T)
    Note: If PVCs occur with a heart rate of less than 60 per minute, the *first* drug to use is atropine, 1 mg IV, followed by isoproterenol as needed.
7 If ventricular tachycardia occurs without loss of pulse or consciousness, give lidocaine bolus, 100 mg I.V. If lidocaine fails, give procainamide. For ventricular tachycardia intractable to both the drugs, give bretylium.
8 Severe sinus tachycardia compromising cardiac output may be suppressed with propranolol.
9 Atrial fibrillation with a rapid ventricular rate should be controlled with digitalis if the patient is conscious and with electrical countershock if the patient is unconscious.

In suspected myocardial infarction with *hypotension* (systolic arterial pressure below 90 mm Hg), i.e. cardiogenic shock, normalize heart rate, control dysrhythmias, and use invasive arterial and pulmonary artery pressure monitoring for titration of hemodynamic life support. With pulmonary artery wedge pressure below 12 mmHg, use 100-200 ml I.V. fluid challenges. Aim for a wedge pressure of 15-18 mmHg for optimal cardiac output. Among vasoactive agents, dopamine is most popular, as it increases cardiac contractility without producing vasoconstriction at infusion rates of 1-10 micrograms/kg per minute. Norepinephrine may be necessary for arterial pressure support. In cases of profound hypotension, assisted circulation by intra-aortic balloon pumping, in addition to cardiac stimulants and vasoconstrictors, may be beneficial (Kantrowitz). This is an expensive, specialized measure requiring an experienced intensive care team. Intra-aortic balloon counterpulsation occasionally can turn the tide in cardiogenic shock, which otherwise is associated with an 80% mortality. The method reduces peripheral resistance during systole and increases diastolic coronary blood flow.

In acute myocardial infarction with *hypertension* (systolic blood pressure above 130 mmHg), attempt to normalize the blood pressure with sublingual nitroglycerin, I.V furosemide or ethancrynic acid and, in an advanced intensive care setting, by titrated I.V. infusion of nitroprusside with arterial pressure monitoring.

In acute *pulmonary edema* associated with acute myocardial infarction, give 100% oxygen by mask, preferably with spontaneous, continuous positive pressure breathing (Chapter 1B). Place the patient into a full upright sitting position with legs dangling dependent; normalize arterial pressure (see above) and give morphine I.V. in titrated doses of 5 mg/70 kg each, to relieve anxiety and tachypnea and to produce «bloodless phlebotomy». Use morphine with caution, so as not to induce severe hypotension. If morphine fails, actual phlebotomy of 500 ml of blood may provide dramatic improvement. Monitor and normalize pulmonary artery wedge pressure if possible. If all this fails and arterial PO_2 cannot be maintained above about 80 mmHg with oxygen by mask, or if foam fills the tracheobronchial tree, then intubate the trachea and control ventilation with PEEP. If necessary use heavy sedation and relaxation.

Miscellaneous Conditions Requiring Resuscitation

In *electric shock* several special considerations apply. Household current may cause ventricular fibrillation. High voltage current passing through the heart causes sustained systole as long as the current flows; and passing through the brain can cause apnea; this results in secondary asphyxial cardiac arrest (asystole), which can be reversed by CPR at the scene. In addition electric shock can cause tissue burns. In general, the procedure for dealing with victims of electric shock is as follows:

Treatment of Victims of Electric Shock

1 Make sure the victim is no longer in contact with the current source!
  a If possible, shut off the current source.
  b Otherwise, dislodge the victim from contact with the current source using a stick, rope, or other nonconductive implement.
2 CPR-ABCs and DEFs (defibrillation) as needed.
3 Special considerations
  a Tetanic muscle spasms may have caused fractures to long bones and damage to spine. Handle the patient accordingly.
  b The magnitude and severity of internal tissue damage cannot be gauged from external burns. Thus, even patients who wake up quickly after electrocution must be hospitalized.

A special instance of electric shock is that which occurs on top of an *electric pole*. If cardiac arrest develops in this situation, deliver a precordial thump and initiate mouth-to-mouth breathing; then lower the victim as rapidly as possible to the ground. CPR is not effective when the victim is in the upright position, for it does not permit adequate venous return, thus the victim should be placed supine with all possible speed.

Hypothermia with cardiac arrest may require thoracotomy or heart-lung machine for rewarming. Cardiac arrest due to *hyperthermia* (heat stroke) is reversible by surface cooling plus standard CPR (Sassano).

In *severe multi-trauma* with *head injury* and coma, the traumatic impact itself can cause instantaneous transient apnea. Resumption of spontaneous breathing movements may be hindered by airway obstruction from lack of head tilt and jaw thrust. Therefore, bystanders at the scene should appreciate and have been trained not only in measures for airway control in such patients — jaw thrust plus moderate backward tilt of the head — but also in mouth-to-mouth or mouth-to-nose breathing. A few minutes after impact, cerebral acidosis usually stimulates spontaneous hyperventilation, and it is this breathing pattern that is usually seen in such patients upon their arrival in the emergency room. Since periods of shallow breathing or aspiration often result in hypoxemia, transport to hospital must be with oxygen inhalation.

In *crushing chest* injury, the patient with a pulse usually requires only oxygen inhalation during transportation. Artificial ventilation outside the hospital should be performed only if absolutely necessary. Pleural drainage equipment should be ready, because of the possibility of provoking tension pneumothorax by positive airway pressure in the presence of lung injury. In the hospital, however, in cases of severe crushing chest injury, prolonged controlled postitive pressure ventilation via tracheostomy tube has become an important therapy (Moerch), not only to counteract the pulmonary shunting, but also to provide internal orthopedic fixation for broken ribs. If the patient with crushed chest develops cardiac arrest, start with closed-chest CPR and switch to open-chest CPR if the closed technique fails to produce a palpable pulse or when uncontrollable intrathoracic hemorrhage is suspected.

In many *other special resuscitative problems* posed by conditions leading to cardiopulmonary failure (e.g., tension pneumothorax, aspiration, status asthmaticus, cardiac tamponade, pulmonary embolism, anaphylactic shock, carbon monoxide poisoning, hypoglycemia), the principles of modern CPR apply (Chapters I—III). Special additional measures required are discussed in the intensive care literature (Shoemaker; Safar, Lawin; Kucher, Weil, Grenvik).

Complications and Pitfalls of CPR
CPR can cause complications, even if performed correctly. Some are minor compared with the certain death if CPR is not started; others leave residual problems. The following are only a few examples.

Backward tilt of the head and positive pressure *inflation attempts* to ventilate the lungs do not by themselves produce serious complications, even in a patient who does not need them, provided they are performed correctly. If the airway is inadequate or inflations are too forceful, however, gastric insufflation may occur and provoke regurgitation and inhalation of gastric contents.

In the aged with atherosclerosis, maximal backward tilt of the head, particularly when the head is turned to the side, can cause circulatory impairment of the vertebral artery-basilar artery system, resulting in brain stem damage. In accident victims, maximal backward head tilt, turning the head to the side, and ante-flexion of the head may all aggravate a spinal cord injury and cause paralysis; thus in these patients, only moderate backward tilt of the head, as part of a triple airway maneuver, is recommended.

External cardiac compressions may result in costochondral separations or multiple rib fractures, especially in elderly patients, even if sternal compressions are performed correctly. This is not necessarily a serious complicaton. Should a flail chest result, prolonged controlled ventilation may be necessary after resuscitation. Pressure applied too high may cause sternal fracture. Pressure applied too low may rupture the liver or cause regurgitation. Pressure applied laterally may fracture ribs, leading to pneumo-or hemothorax or lung contusion. Bone marrow emboli are possible but are not considered to be obstacles to recovery. Every patient after an episode of external cardiac compressions should have a chest X-ray as soon as practically possible.

The recommended initial *stepwise inflation* of the lungs without waiting for full exhalation may reinflate alveoli, but can also increase pharyngeal pressure to such an extent that the stomach becomes distended. Lung rupture with tension pneumothorax is possible when excessive volumes are blown into the lungs of infants or when the patient's lungs are diseased, e.g., in emphysema.

Endotracheal intubation attempts, if prolonged, may produce asphyxia and cardiac arrest. Endotracheal intubation attempts can, as well, aggravate lifethreatening dysrhythmias in the presence of hypoxemia.

Central venous catheter insertions via the *subclavian route* interrupts cardiac compressions and may cause pneumothorax, hemothorax and mediastinal infusion.

The American Heart Association enumerates these *salient points:*

1 Do not interrupt CPR for more than 5 seconds, except for tracheal intubation and moving the victim over stairways. These maneuvers should not exceed 15 seconds each.

2 Do not, under most circumstances, move the patient until he is stabilized; restoring spontaneous circulation at the scene has resulted in higher survival rates than transporting the patient with CPR and restarting spontaneous circulation in the emergency department. (Stabilization includes ventilation, oxygenation, venous lifeline, EKG monitoring, and communication for consultations and arrangement for hospital admission).

There are exceptions to the requirement for stabilization at the scene, where ambulance personnel are not trained or equipped to use the invasive treatment required for such rapidly life-threatening conditions as airway closure by laryngeal edema; tension pneumothorax; pericardial tamponade; intractable heart block requiring pacemaker insertion; hypothermic cardiac arrest requiring warm infusions or thoracotomy; and internal hemorrhage requiring resuscitative surgery. Under such circumstances rapid transportation without prior stabilization and merely life support as feasible is necessary.

3 To avoid injury to the liver, do not maintain pressure on the abdomen to decompress the stomach while CPR is being performed.

4 Pay attention to details of techniques.

Chapter V

TEACHING OF FIRST AID
AND RESUSCITATION

What to Teach to Whom (Table XII)

Providing society with optimal «Life Supporting First Aid and Resuscitation» (i.e., «Life Support»), in order to reduce mortality and morbidity, is conditioned by optimal teaching. The *quality* of teaching aims at providing potential rescuers with the knowledge, skills, reassurance and motivation it takes to make them effective in real life situations. The *quantity* of teaching aims at training enough rescuers to make Life Support immediately available.

Each community, region or country should have an organized system for teaching and testing First Aid and resuscitation knowledge and skills at all levels, ranging from the lay public to physician specialists (Safar, Carveth, Amer. Heart Assoc.).

Table XII summarizes the author's views regarding which personnel groups should learn specific Life Support phases, steps and measures. All of the Basic Life Support and most of the Advanced and Prolonged Life Support techniques listed in Table XII and described in this manual have been subjected to studies that demonstrated their teachability. The recommendations of Table XII may vary with regional differences in personnel qualification levels and may in the future be changed by the introduction of new life support techniques and educational methods.

Guidelines for teaching should be as uniform as possible within each country, at least for the training of nonphysicians, and should hopefully be at least similar (although not necessarily identical) throughout the world. Guidelines regarding which techniques to teach the lay public need to be clearly defined to avoid confusion; guidelines regarding what to teach health care personnel (from life-guards to physician specialists), on the other hand, require more flexibility, to facilitate updating of concepts and techniques as needed.

TABLE XII

What to Teach – to Whom **

● should be taught
○ might be taught
— should not be taught

Phases	Steps	Measures	Lay public	Police, Fireman, Lifeguard	Ambulance attendant, Technician	General nurse	Intensive care nurse, Paramedic	Physician, Medical student, Dentist	Physician specialist
		performed							
I BASIC LIFE SUPPORT – BLS (Emergency oxygenation)	Airway Control	**WITHOUT equipment**							
		* Head tilt	●	●	●	●	●	●	●
		* Supine aligned position	○	●	●	●	●	●	●
		* Stable side position	●	●	●	●	●	●	●
		* Triple airway maneuver (Jaw thrust)	○	○	○	○	●	○	●
		* Manual clearing of mouth and throat	●	○	●	●	●	●	●
		Back blows - manual thrusts	○	○	○	○	○	○	○
		WITH equipment							
		Pharyngeal suctioning	—	—	●	●	●	●	●
		Pharyngeal intubation	—	—	●	●	●	●	●
		Esophageal obturator airway insertion	—	—	○	—	○	○	○
		Endotracheal intubation	—	—	—	—	●	●	●
		Tracheobronchial suctioning	—	—	—	○	●	●	●
		Cricothyrotomy	—	—	—	—	○	○	●
		Translaryngeal O₂ jet insufflation	—	—	—	—	○	○	●
		Tracheotomy	—	—	—	—	—	○	●
		Bronchoscopy	—	—	—	—	—	—	●
		Bronchodilation	—	—	—	○	○	○	●
		Pleural drainage	—	—	—	—	○	○	●

Table — Life Supporting First Aid phases and measures

Breathing Support	
WITHOUT equipment	
* Mouth-to-mouth (nose) ventilation	
WITH equipment	
Mouth-to-adjunct without O_2	
Mouth-to-adjunct with O_2	
Manual bag-mask (tube) O_2 ventilation	
Hand-triggered O_2 ventilation	
Mechanical ventilation	
Circulation Support	
WITHOUT equipment	
* Control of ext. hemorrh.	
* Position for shock	
Pulse checking	
Manual chest compressions	
– single operator	
– two operators	
WITH equipment	
Mechanical chest compression	
Open chest cardiac compression	
Pressure pants (MAST trousers)	
II ADVANCED LIFE SUPPORT – ALS (Restoration of spontaneous circulation)	
Drugs and Fluids — IV Lifeline peripheral / central	
Electrocardiography — EKG monitoring	
Fibrillation Treatment — Defibrillation	
Gauging — Determine and treat cause of demise / Determine salvageability	
III PROLONGED LIFE SUPPORT – PLS (Cerebral resuscitation and post-resuscitation Intensive therapy)	
Human mentation — Cerebral resuscitation	
Intensive care — Multiple organ support	

* Life Supporting First Aid

** Based in part on education research supported by NIH contract # HR 42965

185

The agency responsible for providing guidelines on the teaching of CPCR techniques will have to consider several questions:

1 Does the technique in question have documented life-saving potential?
2 What are the possible risks and complications of the technique, and are these outweighed by the potential benefits?
3 Is the teaching of this technique compatible with local needs and resources?
4 Can the technique be taught, and will the student be able subsequently to employ his skills when the need arises.

Guidelines are indispensable for the successful implementation of large and decentralized teaching programs, whether in hospitals, by organizations or in schools. This manual, written with international validity, contains the necessary subject matter to be considered for the formation of national guidelines.

Teaching the Lay Public
The Need for Mass Training
It has been shown by many investigators that the sooner resuscitation is started after ventilatory or circulatory arrest, the better the chances of survival (Elam, Lind, Lund, Cobb, Safar). Immediate initiation of Life Support measures, which is highly desirable, can, in the majority of cases, be achieved only through action by bystanders. Consequently, there is a need to teach as many people as possible to become efficient resuscitators. Ideally, the whole teachable population should be taught in Life Supporting First Aid and CPR Basic Life Support without equipment (Table XII), because this would yield the highest feasible salvage rates. The documentation to justify this recommendation is so massive that there is now scarcely any justification for rejecting or discouraging this kind of training for the masses on the grounds that it may do more harm than good.

Teaching the lay public mouth-to-mouth ventilation (Lind) and CPR (Cobb) has been proven to save lives. It has also been shown that such teaching is effective (Lind, Winchell, Berkebile, Safar, Breivik, Esposito). Usually, the general lay public should be taught only such measures as they can perform without adjuncts. This limits the contents of learning programs to a reasonable number of techniques and procedures which can be properly learned in a short time. Also it prevents improper use of equipment due to insufficient understanding and practice.

Prerequisites for Mass Training
In the U.S.A. as well as in some other countries, campaigns to teach CPR Basic Life Support to the public have been in progress for some years, and have resulted in the training of millions of people. Heart associations, Red Cross Societies and other humanitarian organizations

have made remarkable efforts in recent years to teach whomever will take courses on a voluntary basis.

In recent years, school systems have also become involved to a noticeable extent. In the future, schools should play an even greater role in the dissemination of First Aid and CPR Basic Life Support proficiency to the public at large. School age is excellent for learning these relatively simple psychomotor skills and the necessary knowledge. Teaching school children also allows for annual retraining, which education research has shown to be important for retaining performance capability. Later in life, those who once received initial training in school, can be retrained during military service or when applying for a driver's license. Some target groups such as high risk industrial workers and family members of cardiac patients can best be taught by voluntary First Aid organizations.

There are large differences between countries in their readiness to start mass training in First Aid and CPR Basic Life Support. In countries where such training has been started on a large scale, the following evolutionary stages have been recognized.

1 Medical consensus. While enthusiasts have promoted CPR training of the general public, conservative members of the medical profession have discouraged liberal dissemination of what they consider professional skills, arguing that in the hands of the lay public these measures might do more harm than good. Today there is scientific documentation of the desirability, feasibility, and safety of teaching Life Supporting First Aid and CPR Basic Life Support without equipment to the entire teachable population. Rejecting or discouraging such teaching is not justified anywhere. Physicians and others who are entitled to an opinion, should be sufficiently well informed about the results of CPR teaching and practice. It is natural that anesthesiologists have taken the leading role as initiators and catalysts. Other authoritative groups of physicians have been cardiologists and surgeons.

2 *Guidelines.* Guidelines for teaching and practicing First Aid and resuscitation can be drawn on a national level, or derived unmodified or modified from another country (e.g., those of the Amer. Heart Assoc.) or from an international organization which represents experts in resuscitation (e.g., the WFSA).

3 *Public awareness.* When the importance of First Aid and resuscitation by bystanders is understood by the public at large, the general response is overwhelmingly positive to accept an active role in life-threatening emergencies. The news media have helped greatly in bringing about such an understanding. For example, a Gallup poll conducted in 1977 in the U.S.A. showed that 65% of the population had heard about CPR, 54% would like to take a CPR course, and 80% would like to make CPR training a requirement for all high school students. This confirms that in 1977 the average American had been

quite well informed and was ready to be involved.

4 *Implementation.* Programs for training and retraining of instructors and rescuers have evolved like the branches of a tree. We recommend that all school children be required to have annual training in Life Supporting First Aid starting at age 11; and CPR Basic Life Support without equipment starting at age 13.

Implementation of training programs will depend upon available training materials and methods and instructors-coordinators (organizers) (see below).

Teaching Health Care Personnel (Table XII)
Basic Life Support

All health care personnel, from first responders, like police, firemen, lifeguards, etc. up to physician specialists, should be trained in Life Supporting First Aid and CPR Steps ABC without equipment. In addition, each category of personnel should be trained in steps and measures that require use of equipment, to a level decided by ability, facilities and needs of that personnel group (Table XII).

In spite of the intensified interest in resuscitation in recent years among non-physician health care personnel, many physicians are still incapable of performing CPR Steps ABC, because their misjudgment of their own capabilities often causes them to avoid further training (Schwartz A). Physicians should reassess their capability and learn those steps of resuscitation which they might need to master in emergencies.

All practicing physicians, dentists, and nurses, including hospital physician house staff and attending staff, should be required to annually demonstrate proficiency in CPR steps ABC with simple equipment items used in the hospital. They can do so by participating in resuscitation efforts on patients, or by passing knowledge and skill tests which may or may not be preceded by a training course.

Advanced and Prolonged Life Support.

Beyond basic life support, all physicians, dentists, nurses, inhalation therapists and paramedical ambulance personnel should learn advanced life support steps according to qualifications. This requires that nurses be permitted to defibrillate and administer drugs as pre-ordered by physicians. In addition, physicians and nurses working in anesthesiology, emergency departments and intensive care units should be trained in some aspects of prolonged life support, including new cerebral resuscitation measures. CPR Basic, Advanced and Prolonged life support should be included in the curricula of all health profession schools. Annual retraining is necessary unless the trainee is frequently involved in actual resuscitation cases.

Teaching Methodology (Table XIII; Fig. 45)
In the late 1950's studies in Baltimore (Safar) demonstrated that lay persons could effectively perform mouth-to-mouth ventilation on anesthetized human volunteers merely after having watched a demonstration or seen pictures. The same seems to be the case for other Life Supporting First Aid measures (Esposito).

When in 1960 the Laerdal Resusci-Anne manikin became available it was shown in Norway that practicing mouth-to-mouth breathing on manikins improved performance (Lind). In 1964, manikin practice was also found to improve correct performance rates and to reduce potentially injurious performance rates of non-physicians after training in CPR Basic Life Support without equipment (Winchell). Since 1960, training programs for external CPR rescuers were developed in the U.S.A. (Jude, Safar, Gordon), in Australia (Brophy) and subsequently in other countries; the first CPR instructors' courses for Basic and Advanced Life Support were developed in Pittsburgh (Safar).

Selected, motivated and qualified non-physicians should receive *instructors' courses* in CPR Basic Life Support without equipment; and selected physicians should receive instructors' courses in the use of equipment and in Advanced Life Support. In some countries, in addition, selected nurse and paramedic instructors have also been trained to teach a variety of Advanced Life Support measures. For the teaching of physicians and nurses in Prolonged Life Support (intensive therapy, including cerebral resuscitation), hospital-based guided patient care experiences are required (Table XIII).

Most CPR courses given by instructors are erroneously limited by time. Individualized learning of knowledge and skills to perfection (i.e., passing tests) is more important than course hours. Also most traditional courses given by instructors include lengthy lectures with slides, which fail to teach the necessary skills. Most important is skill practice on manikins and on one another, coached by the instructor until perfect performance is achieved.

Many persons have already acquired some knowledge and skills in First Aid and resuscitation. Such individuals should not be required to take lengthy courses, but rather should be tested to determine the level of knowledge and skills already acquired. Based on test results, remedial self-training and retesting in specific areas of deficit can be provided before certification.

Teaching methods for Life Support comprise the following 3 elements.
1 *Verbal instruction*
This conveys the knowledge items and provides the necessary guidance of skill practice. Clarity, accuracy and repetition are necessary. In the use of self-teaching systems, instruction can be spoken by the coordinator (preferably learned by heart) or replayed from an audiotape or similar medium, or read by a student.

2 *Visualization*

Techniques and procedures can be visualized in form of demonstrations, blackboard drawings, printed pictures or charts, projected slides, or films. Films made especially for motivational impact are useful for showing prior to training. Good skills-demonstration films are useful as supplements to illustrations, to show specific techniques, preferably in slow motion. Selected films can also be successfully shown after training to broaden the impact of learning.

Illustrations are generally superior to films for the teaching of accuracy of techniques. The illustrations should be correct, simple to understand, and simple to show, preferably without the need for projection equipment. Projected slides are for large audiences.

3 *Practice*

Skill practice is the most important aspect for learning First Aid and resuscitation measures. Training manikins must be used for practicing lung ventilation, chest compression and a number of other steps, whereas some other measures can be practiced effectively on live persons, anesthetized patients, and more rarely, on human corpses and laboratory animals (Table XIII).

Manikins (Fig. 44) should be as realistic as practically feasible to enhance motivation and physiologically correct learning. Each student should have enough time for manikin practice to reach perfection in performance. To obtain this, lecturing should be kept at a minimum, and student groups should be small. Ideally, there should be no more than 4-6 students per manikin for any given session. Supervised manikin practice to perfection allows guidance and evaluation by the instructor while the student is practicing. The stimulus to learn from such «feedback» should not be underestimated.

Automatic guidance from manikins by way of light signals, dials or other indicators is desirable; and is essential for self-training systems. Diagrammatic records of the student's performance give information that can be studied in detail by the student himself, and provide the evaluator with exact objective data. Recording manikins like the widely field-tested and used Laerdal recording Resusci-Anne manikin are extremely valuable.

CPR manikins should simulate airway obstruction with flexion of the neck, and natural chest resistance to lung inflations and chest compressions; permit the performance of jaw thrust and application of face masks without leak; display the adequacy of ventilation and sternal compressions; and have a carotid pulse that can be made to appear and disappear. Programmable manikins for practicing problem solving with Advanced Life Support measures would be desirable, but are not yet available. Arrhythmia manikins are used for defibrillation practice.

Conscious human volunteers have been used for selected aspects of First Aid and resuscitation practice. Control of external hemorrhage (using stick-on wounds moulages) body positioning and splinting are effectively practiced on one another. Exhaled air ventilation cannot be practiced properly on conscious human volunteers, since their airway does not obstruct with flexion of the neck, or the volunteer resists inflation attempts. On the other hand, head-tilt, jaw-thrust, opening the mouth and finger probe (without deep insertion of the finger) can be demonstrated and practiced. Similarly, while sternal compressions should not be carried out on a conscious human subject, students can demonstrate on one another the exact point for application of pressure and the proper hand position.

Unconscious humans, i.e. anesthetized patients, may be used for practicing airway control, various methods of artificial ventilation, cannulation of vessels and monitoring of vital signs. All such activities, however, should be under the strictest control of a staff anesthesiologist who assumes the responsibility for possible injuries. Supervised practice on anesthetized patients, during the time spent with an anesthesia service, is the «ultimate» method for the acquisition of knowledge, judgment and skills with Basic and Advanced Life Support measures (except for sternal compressions which should be practiced on manikins). It is difficult to acquire resuscitation skills under controlled conditions in intensive care units or during hospital-wide resuscitation attempts, as they should be carried out by personnel already skilled in these measures.

Human corpses have been used for practicing resuscitation. In some countries consent from relatives is required. Relaxed fresh corpses are ideal, but usually not available when needed, making training programs which include corpses, difficult to organize. After rigor mortis has set in, corpses are not suitable for practicing most resuscitation techniques, except insertion of an endotracheal tube.

Laboratory animals have been used effectively for the demonstration and practice of certain skills and decision making, such as electrocardiography, defibrillation, drug therapy, open-chest cardiac compressions, intubation, catheterization of vessels and mechanical ventilation. The first open-chest and closed-chest cardiac resuscitation training programs in the 1950's in Baltimore (Safar and Redding) and Cleveland (Beck and Leighninger) included dog laboratory demonstration and practice sessions for physicians and medical students. These sessions proved particularly valuable for demonstrating various patterns of dying, and techniques for restoration of spontaneous circulation. The dog is not suitable, however, for practicing basic life support, because its airway does not reliably obstruct with flexion of the neck; furthermore, mouth-to-mouth ventilation is not aesthetically or practically feasible on the dog, nor can sternal compressions be practiced realistically.. The anterior/posterior diameter of the dog's thorax, in relation to its width, is greater than that of the human.

The unavailability of animal laboratories in hospitals makes it necessary to practice certain steps of Advanced Life Support on the less realistic arrhythmia manikins. These practice sessions should include detailed demonstration and handling of the equipment and supplies on resuscitation carts used in the local hospital.

Self-training systems (Fig. 44) have many advantages over traditional lectures and instructor-coached manikin practice. People learn at individual rates; therefore, training programs should allow for individualized learning to perfection. Self-training systems should encourage students to acquire knowledge from illustrated texts, or tape recorded lectures, or both. Self-training systems have also proven effective for the acquisition of skills in Life Supporting First Aid (Breivik, Esposito) and CPR Basic Life Support (Berkebile, Safar). These systems guide skill practice on manikins or one another through demonstration of pictures (and optional films) and coaching by audiotaped narration or the text of manuals.

Well qualified Life Support instructors are usually scarce, and even the greatest enthusiasts may get bored in the long run by the repetitive nature of this type of teaching. Consequently, self-instructional teaching may be most suitable to implement large scale training programs for the lay public; and to keep up ongoing teaching programs for hospital personnel and other health professionals.

Self-training systems require coordinators for organizing and controlling the learning laboratories. A CPR instructor-coordinator, not necessarily one with training in education, should set up the self-training laboratory, trouble shoot, answer questions, test knowledge and skills, coach to perfect performance by remedial training, retest, certify and recertify periodically.

CPR Basic Life Support Without Equipment
In the 1970s the Laerdal self-training system which consists of flip charts, audiotapes, printed guides, a recording adult manikin and an infant manikin, was modified and found to be as effective as instructor methods in teaching CPR Basic Life Support to lay people (Berkebile) and health care personnel (Safar) (Fig. 44). Self-teaching in fact proved more consistent and better controlled than the traditional lecture method. The same proved to be the case for the Laerdal Life Supporting First Aid self-training system (Breivik, Esposito), the main item of which is a special manual. Merely following instructions in the manual for practice on one another measurably increased First Aid skill performance, although for mouth-to-mouth ventilation, only head tilt and jaw thrust, not lung inflations, were practiced on one another, Manikin practice, however, improved mouth-to-mouth performance rates. The manikin is thus desirable for learning ventilation and essential for learning sternal compressions.

CPR Basic Life Support With Equipment
Use of airways, masks, bags and equipment for oxygen administration, suctioning and tracheal intubation should be taught to health professionals. Each trainee should first study illustrated texts and demonstration films, and then come to suitable learning laboratories with manikins, pictures, audiotapes and the necessary equipment and supplies. Learning the use of oxygen equipment requires the presence of a coordinator to prevent accidents.

Proficiency in Endotracheal Intubation
Learning endotracheal intubation requires practice on manikins as well as on anesthetized patients. The use of human corpses and animals is optional. This author recommends the following training program:

1. Students should study an illustrated text (e.g. Chapter IA of this manual) and then view a good training intubation film, e.g. «Endotracheal Intubation Manikin Practice» (Sladen).
2. Ability to intubate realistic adult and infant manikins can be acquired through self-teaching or supervised practice. Not only correct tube placement is necessary but also correct sequence of steps and timing. Students should be able to intubate the trachea and start lung ventilation within 30 seconds.
3. Once the manikin intubation technique has been mastered, final training should follow, where feasible, in form of supervised practice on anesthetized patients under controlled conditions; or field performance on patients in need of intubation, under «hand-holding» supervision by the ambulance physician. Supervised training of this type should continue until the instructor is convinced that the student demonstrates clearly that he can be permitted to intubate without supervision.

Other methods for tracheal intubation skill practice include the use of monkeys and cats (which are useful for newborn intubation practice) and human corpses. The special technique for rapid «crash» intubation (Sellick, Stept) is dangerous in the hands of the novice. It requires more than practice on manikins, and should be practiced to perfection on patients scheduled for elective anesthesia, whose lives do not depend on the perfect performance of this technique (Chapter 1A).

Advanced Life Support and Prolonged Life Support
Knowledge can be learned from well illustrated teaching texts, and skills of individual life support techniques from demonstration films, and supervised clinical experience of adequate duration. Practice of Advanced Life Support measures in the learning laboratory, if possible, should include dysrhythmia recognition and application of defibrillating electrodes on the arrhythmia manikin or other suitable training aid. If an intravenous infusion manikin is not available, some programs encourage

TABLE XIII

Preferred Training Methods **

● should be taught
○ might be taught
— should not be taught

Phases	Steps	Measures	Manikins	Co-students	Anesth. patients	Human corpses	Lab-animals	Supervised clinical experience
I BASIC LIFE SUPPORT – BLS (Emergency oxygenation)	Airway Control	**WITHOUT equipment**						
		* Head tilt	●	○	●	○	—	●
		* Supine aligned position	○	●	○	○	—	—
		* Stable side position	○	●	○	○	—	●
		* Triple airway maneuver (Jaw thrust)	●	○	●	○	—	○
		* Manual clearing of mouth and throat	●	○	○	○	—	—
		Back blows - manual thrusts	●	○	—	○	—	—
		WITH equipment						
		Pharyngeal suctioning	●	—	○	○	—	○
		Pharyngeal intubation	●	—	○	○	—	●
		Esophageal obturator airway insertion	●	—	○	○	●	○
		Endotracheal intubation	●	—	●	○	●	●
		Tracheobronchial suctioning	●	—	●	○	●	●
		Cricothyrotomy	○	—	—	○	●	—
		Translaryngeal O2 jet insufflation	○	—	—	○	—	—
		Tracheotomy	—	—	—	○	●	●
		Bronchoscopy	●	—	—	○	●	●
		Bronchodilation	—	—	—	—	—	●
		Pleural drainage	—	—	—	○	●	●

Table — Stages and phases of cardiopulmonary-cerebral resuscitation (marks: ● = essential, ○ = optional/adjunct, — = not applicable)

	1	2	3	4	5	6
I — BASIC LIFE SUPPORT						
Breathing Support						
WITHOUT equipment						
* Mouth-to-mouth (nose) ventilation	●	—	—	○	—	●
Mouth-to-mouth hand-head position	●	●	—	○	●	●
WITH equipment						
Mouth-to-adjunct without O_2	●	—	—	○	○	○
Mouth-to-adjunct with O_2	●	—	—	○	○	○
Manual bag-mask (tube) O_2 ventilation	●	—	—	○	○	○
Hand-triggered O_2 ventilation	●	—	—	○	●	●
Mechanical ventilation	○	○	—	○	●	●
Circulation Support						
WITHOUT equipment						
* Control of ext. hemorrh.	○	●	—	—	○	○
* Position for shock	○	●	—	—		●
Pulse checking	●	●	○	—	○	●
Manual chest compressions						
– single operator	●	—	○	—	○	●
– two operators	●	—	○	—	●	●
WITH equipment						
Mechanical chest compression	●	—	○	—	●	●
Open chest cardiac compression	—	—	—	—	●	●
Pressure pants (MAST trousers)	○	○	—	○	—	●
II — ADVANCED LIFE SUPPORT – ALS (Restoration of spontaneous circulation)						
Drugs and Fluids — IV Lifeline peripheral	○	○	—	○	●	●
— central	—	—	—	○	●	●
Electrocardiography — EKG monitoring	○	—	○	—	●	●
Fibrillation Treatment — Defibrillation	○	—	—	—	●	●
III — PROLONGED LIFE SUPPORT – PLS (Cerebral resuscitation and post-resuscitation Intensive therapy)						
Gauging — Determine and treat cause of demise	—	—	—	—	—	●
— Determine salvageability	—	—	—	—	—	●
Human mentation — Cerebral resuscitation	○	○	—	—	●	●
Intensive care — Multiple organ support	○	○	—	—	●	●

* Life Supporting First Aid

** Based in part on education research supported by NIH contract # HR 42965

195

trainees to practice peripheral intravenous infusion on one another. Training objectives, including types and numbers of exposures to clinical problems and performances of treatments, should be clearly defined. Advanced Life Support knowledge and skills should be tested.

Acquisition of knowledge and of judgment in clinical problem solving (e.g., which steps to use in what sequence for restoration of spontaneous circulation) can be enhanced by the use of written or computerized programmed instruction materials (algorithms). For the acquisition of Advanced and Prolonged Life Support skills, no completely effective self-training materials are available yet. There is no substitute for supervised clinical practice. Knowledge of Advanced and Prolonged Life Support, including cerebral resuscitation, *can* be self-learned from teaching texts, without lectures (Safar).

Figure 45: Selected materials for self-training

(A) Car cushion First Aid kit with Life Supporting First Aid manual to teach knowledge and guide skill practice on one another. (For mouth-to-mouth ventilation, manikin practice, B-E, is recommended).

(B) Laerdal's recording Resusci-Anne adult manikin for practicing ventilation and external cardiac resuscitation.

(C) Laerdal's Resusci Baby infant manikin.

(D) Flip charts with pictures; separate sets for Life Supporting First Aid, CPR without equipment, and CPR with equipment.

(E) Cassette player with audiotapes, to be used with flip charts, for coaching, manikin practice.

(F) Manuals for the above, containing same pictures as flip charts and same text as audiotapes.

(G) Manual for instructor and instruction booklet for care of manikin.

(H) Airway and ventilation equipment, including adult, child and infant oropharyngeal airways, nasopharyngeal airways, mouth-to-mouth pocket mask with oxygen nipple, bag-valve-mask unit with oxygen reservoir for adults, children and infants, portable suction with pharyngeal suction tip, and tracheal suction catheter.

(I) Small portable oxygen cylinder with yoke, reducing valve, flowmeter and delivery tube to ventilation and oxygenation equipment (manually triggered oxygen-powered ventilator optional).

(J) Adult and infant intubation manikins with lubricant.

(K) Tracheal intubation equipment and supplies. Stethoscope.

(L) Carrying cases for the above.

Figure 45

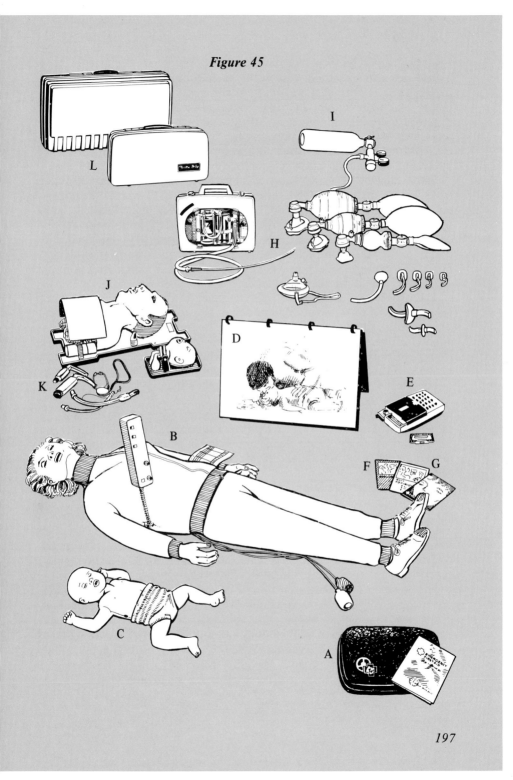

Testing (Tables XIV — XVIII)

Knowledge can be tested reliably by well-designed written tests in the multiple choice format. Each question and answer pair should reflect the material actually taught in the program. For education research, pre-training and post-training tests should have the same questions, with sequences of questions and answers changed. Knowledge *passing criteria* should be established in form of a minimum number of all questions, and all of a few key questions answered correctly.

Skills can be tested reliably during performances which simulate resuscitation attempts, either on manikins (e.g., CPR basic life support; endotracheal intubation), or on human volunteers (e.g., head-tilt, jaw-thrust, hand positions, hemorrhage control, body positioning). At the conclusion of self-learning CPR Basic Life Support on the recording manikin, the trainee produces the record which the examiner evaluates. For skills not practiced on or recorded by the manikin, appropriate checklists should be used (Table XIV — XVIII).

The *criteria* for *passing* skill performance tests should be established on the basis of physiologic requirements for successful resuscitation; and practical considerations, which may call for more lenient criteria to be applied in the testing of lay personnel and more stringent criteria in the testing of health care personnel (Winchell, Berkebile, Amer. Heart Assoc.). For skill testing and certifying copy Tbls. XIV-XVIII.

For the training of millions in Life Supporting First Aid, testing and certifying is impractical and probably not necessary. However, testing for CPR Basic Life Support without equipment is desirable, because of the possibility of causing harm with sternal compressions when they are not needed. Testing of knowledge and skills in the use of equipment and in Advanced and Prolonged Life Support is recommended before certification.

Certification in Life Supporting First Aid should be for the completion of a training program (without obligatory tests). Certification in CPCR should be for the successful completion of defined knowledge and skill tests. Resuscitators and instructors-coordinators should be certified separately; each separately for CPR Basic-, Advanced-, and Prolonged-Life Support (Table XII-XVIII). One cannot (and therefore should not) certify the ability to perform CPR effectively when called upon.

The Resuscitation Research Center of the University of Pittsburgh is preparing a WFSA-sponsored course for CPCR instructors-coordinators, using this manual to convey the required body of knowledge, and emphasizing the use of self-training systems. For information write to Dr. P. Safar, 3434 Fifth Avenue, Pittsburgh, PA 15260 U.S.A.; or to Dr. J. Zorab, Frenchay Hospital, Bristol, U.K.

TABLE XIV

Skill Test on Adult Manikin
Check List and Passing Criteria
For CPR Basic Life Support Without Equipment on Adults
(Adapted from Amer. Heart Assoc.)

Student's name	Date	Evaluator's name

☐ Passed   ☐ Failed

INITIAL PHASE

Measures	Technique	Time
✓ Check if correct sequence	✓ Check if correct performance	✓ Check if within correct time lapse min. - max.

Measures	Technique	Time
1 ☐ Establishing unresponsiveness	☐ Shake shoulder gently / Shout: How are you? / ☐ Call «help»	sec. ☐ 3-5
	☐ Turn patient onto back if found in other position	☐ 3-5
2 ☐ Opening airway	☐ Head tilt-neck lift or ☐ Head tilt-chin support	☐ 3-5
☐ Establishing breathlessness	☐ Keep ear over mouth and nose and observe chest (look-listen-feel)	
3 ☐ Providing initial inflations	☐ 3-5 times, to make chest rise	☐ 3-5
4 ☐ Establishing pulselessness	☐ Palpation of the carotid pulse on near side. Maintain head tilt	☐ 5-10
☐ Activating EMS system	☐ Knows EMS phone No.	
5 ☐ Providing one-rescuer ventilation-compression	☐ Four full cycles providing a total of 60 compressions and 8 ventilations / ☐ Proper rescuer posture / ☐ Landmark checking each time / ☐ Proper hand position / ☐ Proper compression depth (4-5 cm) / ☐ No bouncing. 50/50 compr./relax. / ☐ Proper compressions minute rate (80) / ☐ Adequate ventilation volume (0.8 l) / ☐ Proper ratio vent.-compression (2:15)	☐ 55-65
6 ☐ Checking return of spontaneous pulse and breathing	☐ Feel for carotid pulse / ☐ Check for breathing	☐ 3-5

CONSECUTIVE PHASE

Pass criteria: (A variation of ∓ 10% is permissible)

A single rescuer procedes as above and should perform at least 12 adequate ventilations and 60 correct compressions during initial 100 sec.

When a *second rescuer* becomes available, two rescuer performance should provide 12 ventilations and 60 compressions per minute. Compressions should be given in an uninterrupted rhythm. One ventilation should be interposed between each five compressions.

Takeover and switching of 2 rescuers should be as described in chapter I C.

TABLE XV

Skill Test on Infant Manikin

Check List and Passing Criteria
For CPR Basic Life Support Without Equipment on Infants
(Adapted from Amer. Heart Assoc.)

Student's name	Date	Evaluator's name

☐ Passed   ☐ Failed

INITIAL PHASE

Measures	Technique	Time
✓ Check if correct sequence	✓ Check if correct performance	✓ Check if within correct time lapse min. - max.

1 ☐ Establishing unresponsiveness	☐ Shake shoulder gently ☐ Shout ☐ Call «help» ☐ Turn if necessary	sec. ☐ 3-5
2 ☐ Opening airway ☐ Establishing breathlessness	☐ Moderate head tilt ☐ Keep ear over mouth and nose and observe chest (look-listen-feel)	☐ 3-5
3 ☐ Providing initial inflations	☐ Ventilate 3-5x to make chest rise (rapidly and with small volume)	☐ 3-5
4 ☐ Establishing pulselessness	☐ Palpation of the brachial or femoral pulse on near side	☐ 5-10
☐ Activating EMS system	☐ Knows EMS phone No.	
5 ☐ Providing one-rescuer ventilation-compression	☐ Ten full cycles providing a total of 10 ventilations and 50 compressions ☐ Proper finger position on midsternum ☐ Proper compression depth (1-2 cm) ☐ Proper compression rate/min. (80-100) ☐ Small interposed ventilation volume ☐ Proper ratio compression - vent. (5:1)	☐ 30
6 ☐ Checking return of spontaneous pulse and breathing	☐ Feel for brachial or femoral pulse ☐ Check for breathing	☐ 3-5

CONSECUTIVE PHASE

Pass criteria: (A variation of ∓ 10% is permissible)

The rescuer should during the initial 60 sec. provide at least 45 compressions and 12 ventilations.

200

TABLE XVI

Skill Test on Adult Manikin

Check List and Passing Criteria
For CPR Steps ABC with Equipment
(RRC, Univ. Pittsburgh)

Student's name   Date   Evaluator's name

☐ Passed

☐ Failed

Measures	Technique	Time
	☑ Check if correct performance	☑ Check if within correct time lapse

Measures	Technique	Time
		sec.
Suctioning (CPR recording manikin)	☐ Assembled and tested correctly Suctioning equipment ☐ Demonstrated correct oropharyngeal suctioning	☐ < 45
Pharyngeal intubation (adult intubation manikin)	☐ Inserted correctly oropharyngeal airway ☐ Inserted correctly nasopharyngeal airway	☐ < 15 ☐ < 15
O₂ delivery system (connect to ventilation devices below)	☐ Tightened cylinder yoke before opening valve ☐ Established correct connections to the 3 ventilation devices below ☐ Provided O₂ flow of 5-15 l/min to mask and bag	
Ventilation devices (CPR recording manikin)	☐ Mouth-to-mouth pocket mask Ventilated with at least 3 tidal volumes of 0.8 l ☐ Bag-valve-mask Ventilated with at least 3 tidal volumes of 0.8 l ☐ Manually triggered O₂ ventilator Ventilated with at least 3 tidal volumes of 0.8 l	☐ < 30 ☐ < 30 ☐ < 30

TABLE XVII

Skill Test on Intubation Manikins

Check List and Passing Criteria
For Endotracheal Intubation Manikin Tests
(RRC, Univ. Pittsburgh)

Student's name	Date	Evaluator's name

☐ Passed

☐ Failed

Measures	Technique	Time
	☑ Check if correct performance	☑ Check if within correct time lapse

Measures	Technique	Time
Endotracheal intubation of *adult* manikin	☐ Checked laryngoscope light before use	sec.
	☐ Checked tube patency before use	
	☐ Held laryngoscope correctly	
	☐ Used no grossly traumatic maneuver during intubation attempt	
	☐ Inserted tube into trachea rapidly	☐ < 30
	☐ Gave first lung inflation rapidly via tube by bag-valve or mouth	☐ < 60
	☐ Inflated cuff of tube correctly (with helper)	
	☐ Used bite-block, secured tube and connected ventilation device correctly	
	☐ Checked to rule out bronchial intubation	
Endotracheal intubation of *infant* manikin	☐ Checked laryngoscope light before use	
	☐ Checked tube patency before use	
	☐ Held laryngoscope correctly	
	☐ Used no grossly traumatic maneuver during intubation attempt	
	☐ Inserted tube into trachea rapidly...........	☐ < 30
	☐ Gave first lung inflation rapidly via tube (by mouth)	☐ < 60
	☐ Used bite-block, secured tube and connected ventilation device correctly	
	☐ Checked to rule out bronchial intubation	
Endotracheal suctioning (curved-tipped catheter)	☐ Used correct technique to suction each lung separately	☐ < 60

TABLE XVIII

Skill Test with Advanced Life Support Materials

Check List and Passing Criteria
For Miscellaneous Advanced Life Support Measures
(RRC, Univ. Pittsburgh)

| Student's name | Date | Evaluator's name |

☐ Passed

☐ Failed

Measures	Technique	Time
	☑ Check if correct performance	☑ Check if within correct time lapse

---

Venous infusion
☐ Assembled correctly intravenous infusion and cannulation equipment

☐ Described correctly sites and techniques of peripheral vein cannulation
☐ Described correctly sites and techniques of central vein cannulation

Drugs
☐ Prepared correctly single-dose IV injection of lidocaine for PVCs (pt. with pulse)
☐ Prepared correctly single-dose IV injection of epinephrine (pt. with cardiac arrest)
☐ Prepared correctly single-dose IV injection of bicarbonate (first «blind» dose for pt. with cardiac arrest)

EKG recognition
(arrhythmia manikin)
☐ Applied correctly peripheral EKG electrodes
☐ Applied correctly chest defibrillator-EKG monitor electrodes
☐ Recognized *lethal* EKG patterns (ventric. fibrill., ventric. tachycardia, electric asystole, electromechanical dissociation) .... ☐ 15 sec each
Recognized *life-threatening* EKG patterns .... ☐ 15 sec each

☐ Regular sinus rhythm with multifocal PVCs
☐ Second degree heart block
☐ Third degree heart block

Defibrillation
(arrhythmia manikin,
hospital crash cart)
☐ Charged defibrillator with 200-400 Watt sec.
☐ Placed 2 defibrillating chest electrodes with saline pads correctly   ☐ < 60 sec
☐ Checked for VF before countershock.
☐ Discharged defibrillator and kept paddles on chest to check EKG. Ordered «hands off» before shock
☐ Checked pulse and continued CPR according to EKG rhythm displayed by examiner

203

Chapter VI

ORGANIZATION

Hospital-wide Organization

CPR services inside hospitals that should be in readiness 24 hours per day include: (a) advanced life support capability in the emergency department, ICUs and other special care units, provided by personnel of these units; (b) a hospital-wide resuscitation team response within seconds of calls from anywhere in the hospital, to include critical care units when their staff needs help; and (c) a mechanism for prevention of cardiac arrest and providing life support in myocardial ischemia and infarction, in cases not requiring resuscitation (dysrhythmia recognition and control).

Every acute care hospital should have a specific multi-disciplinary committee with responsibility for providing CPR services 24 hours per day and for ensuring high standards of resuscitation and intensive therapy. This committee may be composed of an anesthesiologist, a cardiologist, a surgeon, a nurse, an administrator, and physician representation of the emergency department and ICU. The committee should be responsible for providing: (1) written treatment protocols; (2) training and practice sessions in CPR; (3) training in intensive therapy; and (4) periodic review of records of resuscitation attempts, with identification of mistakes and feedback to the medical personnel involved, as a means of minimizing the commission of the same mistakes in the future.

Every general hospital with acute care facilities should provide an advanced life support unit in its emergency department so that any patient who has symptoms suggestive of myocardial infarction or other cardiopulmonary emergencies will be placed immediately on monitoring and surveillance, until a definite decision is made regarding his management. If there is a strong suspicion that the patient has had an acute myocardial infarction he should be transferred to the coronary care unit or ICU. During transfer he should be connected to a battery operated monitor-defibrillator. If necessary, appropriate drugs should be administered en route.

Organization and mobilization of hospital personnel for CPR calls will depend on local circumstances. One (usually chaotic) method is a *general response*, i.e., to have all physicians and nurses who hear the alert respond to it. The physician present who is most experienced in resuscitation (which is often difficult to determine or agree upon) must take charge, since lack of team leadership is the most common cause of ineffective, incompetently carried out CPR efforts. The team leader must define the responsibilities of those personnel who are needed and dismiss those who are not. The presence of too many medical personnel at a resuscitation can be as detrimental to the patient's care as the presence of too few.

Another plan is to use a *designated team response*. In this system, the committee appoints a team leader, who exercises decisive team leadership. In large hospitals with 24-hour coverage by physicians of various disciplines, members of one discipline can be chosen on the basis of their experience and availability to assume the role of team leader. This avoids the confusion which occurs at the scene when one discipline is not clearly in charge. The team usually is composed of an anesthesiologist, internist, and surgeon; a crash cart technician or respiratory therapist; and at least two nurses from the arrest location. One potential problem with the designated team leader approach is variability in training and experience of house staff of various departments serving on the CPR team.

In emergency rooms and ICUs, team function occurs automatically, as most members are working together most of the time on non-emergency cases. Lack of skilled, knowledgeable team leadership (because of departmental territorialism), delegation of CPR efforts to inexperienced house staff, involvement of excessive numbers of personnel, and a declining involvement of anesthesiologists with special resuscitation skills in the resuscitation efforts outside the operating rooms, all have led to a deterioration of the quality of CPR efforts in many hospitals, particularly outside of special care units. This trend must be reversed.

The hospital resuscitation team should be capable of performing all phases of CPR, basic and advanced life support, with and without equipment. One method of team function is as follows: The person recognizing the emergency starts resuscitation and calls for a helper, who in turn calls the telephone operator by a pre-arranged alert number that overrides all other calls. The telephone operator pages the team by an emergency code and gives the location. This is essential to avoid delay caused by calling back for the location. The team members respond to the alert and rush to the scene. The team leader takes over ventilation or checks the adequacy of ventilation started by another person and monitors the effectiveness of chest compressions. The cart technician who has brought the crash cart to the scene prepares the defibrillation-EKG monitoring paddles and later attaches the EKG limb electrodes. One nurse assists with intravenous infusion and draws up medications. The second nurse keeps records. The team leader reads the EKG, determines drug therapy, and applies countershocks as needed. If help is scarce, he will insert the intravenous cannula or perform a cut-down. Intubation should be attempted by a staff member who is skilled in the technique and who can perform it quickly. Special nurses, particularly those assigned to the emergency department and ICUs, should be trained and authorized to defibrillate and give special drugs, as preordered.

The patient should be transported from the scene of the resuscitation to the ICU only after he has been stabilized. The person who initiates emergency resuscitation must ensure that the patient receives post-resuscitative intensive care. If complex post-resuscitative intensive care (e.g., brain resuscitation) is indicated, hospitals without this expertise available should seek advice by phone rather than transfer patients from one hospital to another at a time when every minute of sophisticated life support counts.

Community-wide Organization (Table XIX)
CPCR capability must be part of all components of the emergency medical services (EMS) delivery system (Table XIX) (Safar, Frey, Seeley, Amer. Soc. of Anesthesiologists). This makes it an «Emergency and Critical Care Medicine» (ECCM) system. Such a system is only as good as its weakest component. Knowledgeable, authoritative coordination of the system is essential. This can be accomplished either through the voluntary community council approach used in the USA or through local or regional governments as in many other countries.

Each regional system must be coordinated by an *emergency medical operations and communications center,* staffed by experienced paramedical dispatchers who are supported via radio-telephone by ECCM-experienced physicians. The function of this center is to appraise and respond to everyday medical emergencies, as well as major disasters, by mobilizing resources outside hospitals and controlling the flow of patients to hospitals. The center, all ambulance and rescue vehicles, and all emergency hospitals should be linked by two-way radio-telephones. The center should be empowered in each case to select ambulance services and hospitals according to the needs of the patients.

A single public access *telephone number* must be available to reach the dispatching center for emergency medical services. The center should be staffed by personnel capable of identifying the need for basic or advanced life support ambulances, fire department, police or rescue services.

The graded response of community-wide life support should start with education of the *lay public* in life supporting first aid (Breivik, Esposito) and CPR basic life support (Winchell, Berkebile). This could save thousands of lives in many countries each year (Cobb, Lund, Hossli).
Ambulances
All ambulances should be staffed and equipped for basic life support capability by especially trained emergency medical technicians (EMT, EMT I) (basic ambulance personnel). Where there are basic life support personnel only, however, salvage rates of cardiac arrest victims have been disappointing. Therefore, selected ambulances should be upgraded to advanced life support capability through staffing with paramedics (EMT II), nurses or physicians (mobile ICUs).

Prehospital advanced life support was pioneered in the '60s by

TABLE XIX

Community-wide Emergency and Critical Care Medicine System

Components	Service Componenets		Coordination
	Suggested Physician Responsibilities		
	Emergency Dpt. Physicians	CCM (ICU) Physicians	ED plus CCM Physicians
(1) Treatment at the scene recognition of the emergency and aid by bystanders*	—	—	
(2) Initiation of system by bystander**	(+)	—	
(3) Resuscitation and stabilization at the scene by members of the system*	+	(+)	(8) Organization, Communication (9) Planning, Education Evaluation
(4) Transportation with life support* Preferably by advanced life support ambulance service	+	(+)	(10) Research
(5) Treatment in the emergency dpt. multi-disciplinary team team leadership	+ Clinical Base of ED physician	(+) Resus. only	
(6) Management in the operating room by surgeons and anesthesiologists	—	(+)	
(7) Treatment in the ICU Major emergency hospital with advanced physician-staffed ICUs	—	+ Clinical Base of CCM Physician	

Ideally (utopian?) the same group of resuscitologists would be responsible for *all* components (Safar, Lust).

*Prehospital physician advice and radio control of EMT's and paramedics. Presence of physician optional
**Call Mobile ICU ambulance, by universal emergency telephone number.
+ Required; (+) optional
For abbreviations, see Glossary

(from P. Safar 1966, 1973)

physician-staffed ambulances in Czechoslovakia (Sefrna), the Soviet Union (Negovsky), Germany (Frey, Dortman, Ahnefeld) and Ireland (Pantridge). In the U.S.A. these services have evolved later as mobile ICUs (Safar) staffed by specially trained paramedics (Benson) who are under continuous radio command from physicians (Nagel, Cobb, Caroline). There are no outcome data available that clearly favor one staffing pattern over the other.

Advanced life support capability can be achieved even by paramedics with little educational background, as well as part-time volunteers, provided there is strong direction by physicians (Benson, Caroline). Training of advanced life support personnel should include standing orders and treatment protocols based on national standards (Caroline). Non-physicians should be in radio contact with ECCM physicians (Caroline). Most EMS leaders recommend the most cost effective staffing of mobile ICU ambulances. If they are staffed by paramedics, those should be thoroughly trained by physicians in advanced life support, and deliver treatments according to their training and standing orders for which the service's physician director is responsible. These standing orders should be modified by physician guidance via radio as needed. The degree to which paramedics should be permitted to act on their own in resuscitation cases depends on their competence and that of the physician giving the radio command (Nagel, Caroline, Baskett).

The physician director who is knowledgeable and skilled in the management of basic and advanced CPR must assume the medical responsibility for each basic or advanced life support ambulance service. His responsibilities include quality control of patient care and the direct or remote supervision of the activities of paramedical personnel under his command (Caroline). Paramedics must be familiar with the use of voice and EKG telemetry equipment for advanced cardiac care (Nagel). Special continuing education programs for all life support unit staff are required. Non-physician staff (paramedics and nurses) of fixed advanced life support units (see below) must have constant access to radio communication with the physician director — for example the one staffing the EMS operations center. Direction of advanced emergency cardiac care by paramedics and nurses in the field can be enhanced by the optional use of EKG telemetry (Nagel). This method, however, after use in a transition period, has been given up by most ambulance services. The medical director should establish a sound referral policy to have patients delivered to the most appropriate hospital.

Medical control over the EMS system and *pre-hospital* emergency care, both basic and advanced, requires the authority of a specifically assigned physician (medical director), who is responsible for medical care provided by all personnel in the system; this physician must also take responsibility for training, certification, approval of medical equipment and supplies, approval of treatment protocols, and maintenance of quality control, which includes ongoing case reviews. *Pre-hospital advanced life support is the practice of medicine* and therefore must be carried out by physicians or be under continuing direction of physicians with experience in emergency and resuscitative care, who use standing orders and radio command to guide non-physicians. Physicians giving radio command should adhere as much as possible to agreed treatment protocols, to provide some uniformity in the delivery of care, and to improve the standard of care (Caroline).

When trained lay bystanders start CPR at the scene within 4 minutes of cardiac arrest, and advanced life support ambulance personnel subsequently restart spontaneous circulation before reaching the hospital, cerebral recovery rates of over 50% have been achieved among victims of prehospital sudden cardiac death (Lund, Cobb, Crampton, Nagel). In addition experiences in recent wars have shown that with control of hemorrhage at the scene and rapid transportation to an advanced life support surgical facility, if necessary by aircraft, mortality is measurably reduced among victims of severe trauma. Therefore, ideally, each community should provide basic life support outside hospitals within 3 to 4 minutes, and advanced life support within 10 minutes in urban and 30 minutes in rural areas. Realistically, however, it is recognized that this goal cannot be reached in many regions of the world.

When the call suggests respiratory distress, unconsciousness, pulselessness, severe trauma or suspicion of heart attack, the mobile ICU should be dispatched. In many communities a two-stage response has proved practical, i.e., all calls are answered by ambulances providing basic life support; and in cases possibly requiring advanced life support, a mobile ICU or a physician with special equipment in a normal car, arrives at the scene separately. The basic life support ambulance may be used for transporting the patient to the hospital, accompanied by the physician.

The use of *helicopters* or fixed-wing aircraft for the transport of acutely ill and injured patients, from isolated or otherwise inaccessible sites and from smaller hospitals to major emergency hospitals, should be developed (Frey). Heliports should be established at major emergency hospitals close enough to the emergency department to obviate the need for transfer between helicopter and hospital special care unit by ambulance. Helicopter ambulances and fixed-wing aircraft for patient transport should have the same equipment as recommended for mobile ICU-type ambulances.

Hospitals

Life-threatening emergencies, particularly resuscitation cases, should be taken to the nearest hospital that has comprehensive emergency facilities. These major emergency hospitals should be established on a regional basis. They should be staffed around-the-clock by teams of specialists available within minutes and should conform to the highest standards attainable within the community. Unless the patient is beginning to wake up at the scene or during transportation, it is desirable to transfer resuscitation cases to advanced hospital ICUs. Patients suspected of myocardial infarction should be admitted to the nearest hospital that can provide emergency cardiac care.

The ECCM capability of a hospital should be made known to the medical community and the public by designating the hospital as (1) Major (advanced) emergency hospital; (2) Emergency hospital; or (3) basic emergency facility — or some similar categorization. Facility (3) should have an ICU with basic intensive medical care; i.e., full-time of an advanced life support station, at least in the emergency department, but does not have to provide long-term intensive therapy. Hospital (2) should have an ICU with basic intensive medical care; i.e., full-time staffing with specially trained nurses, a (part-time) ICU physician director and coverage by physicians from outside the ICU. Category (1) hospital, usually a «tertiary referral facility» should receive directly from the field cases of multi-trauma and other major life-threatening emergencies with multiple organ failure; the category (1) hospital should have an advanced ICU, staffed around-the-clock with full-time physicians trained or in training in CCM, and directed by a physician with special expertise and interest in CCM.

Disaster Plan

Each regional EMS delivery system and each emergency hospital should have a plan for expanding its resuscitative and surgical capability including radio communications, in case of disasters with large numbers of casualties. The special field of disaster medicine which has so far been primarily the domain of traumatology, restorative surgery, Public Health and rehabilitation, should receive more input from resuscitology (Frey, Club of Mainz). When in a disaster the resources of the regional EMS response system are expected to become exhausted, nationwide and international relief should be sought immediately. This often must rely heavily on modern aircraft delivered medical help and rescue, particularly with helicopters, if extrication and resuscitation (particularly treatment of shock at the scene and rapid transport for resuscitative surgery) are to occur before irreversible vital organ failure or infection has begun. There must be combined medical-logistic authority at the disaster site. Collaboration of civilian agencies and armed forces of various countries is a dream for the future.

Advanced Life Support Units

Advanced life support units (resuscitation units) may be (1) *hospital based* in emergency departments, ICUs or coronary care units; or (2) *outside hospitals* — as (a) *stationary* units («life support station») in special locations such as airports; or (b) *mobile* units in form of special ambulances (mobile ICUs). Widespread basic life support capability of trained members of the lay public and first responders (e.g., policemen, firemen, life guards) should sustain life while calling and waiting for a mobile ICU or transporting the patient to a fixed advanced life support unit.

All these units must be capable of providing basic and advanced life support. The stationary unit should be located in airports, railroad stations, sport arenas, convention centers, stadiums, civic auditoriums, industrial plants, large office building complexes and other areas with large in-transit populations. Mobile ICU ambulances staffed by paramedics can be used as stationary life support units parked temporarily at a special event.

These life support units should be able to provide advanced life support by: (1) identifying patients with cardiopulmonary emergencies; (2) administering oxygen, instituting immediate monitoring, establishing an I.V. infusion prior to obtaining a detailed history; (3) providing continued surveillance until a professional decision on management is made; (4) stabilizing the patient's condition prior to transfer to the hospital; and (5) following guidelines on referrals, record keeping, and communication (American Heart Association).

Advanced life support units should be accessible, clearly marked, and staffed at all times by a team including at least two persons trained in advanced life support, if possible one being a physician. In the absence of a physician, the non-physician personnel should be linked by two-way radio communication with a physician familiar with the unit and its standing orders. The unit must be equipped for rendering basic and advanced life support (Fig. 1, Table I), including the use of equipment, for a variety of emergencies, ranging from severe trauma to sudden cardiac arrest; from infants to adults.

Each unit must have an established referral policy (transfer agreement) to bring the patient to the most appropriate hospital, with life support continuing during transportation.

The equipment, drugs and records required for advanced life support are basically similar whether that life support is carried out within the hospital in a fixed life support station or a mobile ICU. Personnel working in mobile units, however, require additional training, since the special constraints of the work necessitates expertise in communications, EKG telemetry (optional), rescue, extrication, emergency driving, security, local geography and crowd control. Furthermore, *physicians guiding mobile ICU personnel should themselves have first-hand experience in providing advanced life support on the streets and in the field.* (Safar, Caroline).

Equipment for hospital-based, stationary and mobile advanced life support units should at least include basic ingredients of a hospital crash cart. For intra-hospital units, such crash carts should be provided in strategic locations, such as the emergency department, ICU, coronary care unit, operating suite, recovery room, X-ray department, cardiac catheterization laboratory, etc. — and at least one cart should be mobile for hospital-wide use. Each hospital nursing station or floor should have this equipment available for use within 1 to 2 minutes. Ideally, not only mobile ICU ambulances but also ambulances staffed by basic life support personnel should carry advanced life support equipment, in case physicians or paramedics come to the scene and need it.

EQUIPMENT FOR FIXED AND MOBILE LIFE SUPPORT STATIONS

1 **Equipment for CPR steps A and B (Chpts IA, IB):**
   a. oropharyngeal and nasopharyngeal airways of all sizes (S-tubes optional) (Fig. 11)
   b. suction equipment (Fig. 10)
   c. tracheal intubation equipment (Fig. 13)
   d. cricothyrotome (Fig. 16)
   e. translaryngeal oxygen jet insufflation set (optional) (Fig. 17)
   f. mouth-to-mouth pocket mask with oxygen nipple (Fig. 22)
   g. bag-valve-mask unit with oxygen reservoir (Fig. 23)
   h. nasogastric tubes
   i. oxygen supply, at least in the form of two small (size E) cylinders with reducing valve and delivery tube, capable of supplying at least 15 liters of oxygen per minute (Fig. 24).
   j. for life supporting first aid, additional pressure bandages, scissors, tape and sheet (blanket)

2 **Equipment for CPR step C and Advanced Life Support (Chpts IC, II):**
   a. backboard for CPR
   b. folded towels
   c. battery powered (portable, direct current) defibrillator with EKG monitor oscilloscope. EKG electrodes incorporated into the external defibrillator paddles. EKG needle and stick-on electrodes
   d. sterile internal defibrillator paddles for adults and children
   e. thoracotomy tray for open-chest CPR
   f. pleural drainage set
   g. sterile gloves
   h. blood pressure cuff and stethoscope
   i. venous tourniquets
   j. adhesive tape
   k. scissors
   l. bladder catheterization set

m. portable EKG recorder with connection to the defibrillator - EKG monitor, with chest leads for refined EKG diagnosis (optional)

n. IV infusion sets with normal and micro-drips, including catheter-inside and catheter-outside needles (plastic cannulae) sizes 14 to 22 gauge (including long CVP catheters and CVP manometer)

o. infusion stopcocks and extension tubes

p. IV solutions in plastic bags, including
   (1) 5 percent dextrose
   (2) Ringer's or isotonic sodium chloride solution
   (3) 5 percent dextrose in 0.5 percent sodium chloride
   (4) colloid solutions, such as dextran, hydroxyethyl starch and/or 5 percent albumin in saline

q. for the administration of drugs, an assortment of syringes (and needles) and a long intracardiac needle

r. cervical collar, spine board (long and short), splints

3 Recommended Drugs (Chpt II):
   a. epinephrine
   b. sodium bicarbonate
   c. norepinephrine
   d. dopamine
   e. a vasodilator (e.g., nitroprusside, trimethaphan, chlorpromazine)
   f. thiopental or pentobarbital;diazepam
   g. succinylcholine
   h. pancuronium
   i. lidocaine
   j. procainamide
   k. bretylium
   l. atropine
   m. diphenylhydantoin
   n. methylprednisolone or dexamenthasone
   o. furosemide or ethacrynic acid
   p. mannitol
   q. morphine
   r. digoxin
   s. lanatoside or strophantin
   t. calcium chloride
   u. dextrose 20 %
   v. metaraminol
   w. isoproterenol
   x. aminophylline
   y. metaproterenol aerosol
   z. antihistamine

aa. maloxone (Narcan)

bb. other drugs, depending on personal preference.

Prefilled syringes ready for injection are desirable. Individual-dose vials are preferred over mutiple-dose vials.

Legal Considerations

Medico-legal recommendations concerning CPR remain in flux, since the law follows rather than precedes events occurring in practice and precedents set by law suits after injury. Laws vary greatly between states and countries. CPCR practitioners, teachers and organizers should familiarize themselves with existing laws relevant to resuscitation in their own region, such as the Medical Practice Act, the Good Samaritan Act, definition of death and «living will» for the right to die without senseless resuscitation efforts. The views presented here are mostly those of the American Heart Association CPR Committee legal advisers.

Fear of the law is unjustified. In the USA there has never been a case of a successfully pursued lawsuit for resuscitation performed in the field even if it resulted in an undesirable outcome. There have been, however, many lawsuits won by patients' relatives when in hospitals failure to attempt resuscitation has led to injury or death.

Legal advisors state that standards and guidelines for CPR do not intend to limit or inhibit persons inside or outside hospitals from providing emergency medical treatment. Since it may be unrealistic to expect immediate compliance with these standards in some circumstances, a reasonable time for implementation should be allowed. For legal considerations of initiation and termination of resuscitation efforts and orders not to resuscitate, see Chapter III.

State laws should clarify what non-physician health care personnel can and should do; clarify the medical practice act accordingly; give immunity (for acts done in good faith and not involving gross negligence or willful, wanton, or reckless misconduct) for those certified in basic or advanced life support; make training and certification in CPR a job requirement for key health care personnel; and prevent law enforcement officers from interferring with resuscitation efforts by qualified persons. Ideally, hospitals should establish regulations to restrict hospital physician staff privileges to those who have shown the ability to render basic life support.

In most regions, there are several general laws relevant to the provision of emergency life support measures. The doctrine of «res ipsa loquitur» (The thing speaks for itself) can be explained by the example of a cardiac arrest in the operating room in which it might be assumed that negligence occurred, and that the professional must explain that negligence did not occur. The «Good Samaritan Law», in force in most of the United States and other countries, is meant to protect medical and paramedical persons from civil liability when, acting in good faith, they attempt to resuscitate a person. This includes the physician who renders help at the scene outside the hospital or walks into a hospital and is suddenly called upon to help. «Informed consent» applies to surgical and other therapeutic procedures that may result in cardiac arrest or indeed in any untoward and undesirable result. It has been shown to be impossible to state specifically what «informed consent» should include. In general, there is no substitute for good communication between physician and patient or, if the patient is unconscious, his relatives. Informed consent cannot be obtained in resuscitation cases when the patient is unconscious, the relatives are not available or in emotional shock, and special (often innovative) operative or otherwise invasive treatments are needed immediately in order to be effective. For these situations the «emergency exception» for informed consent applies. This exception should apply also to well designed and peer-reviewed clinical resuscitation research protocols (Abramson).

Hospitals and ambulance services must live up to the standards of care and practice in the community. If a hospital or ambulance service lacks appropriate equipment and/or resuscitation procedures, it can be held liable for falling below this standard. Community standards are increasingly interpreted by law as accepted practices beyond the local level, even at national and international levels.

CONCLUSIONS

The phases and steps of cardiopulmonary-cerebral resuscitation represent the *sine qua non* of knowledge and skills required of emergency and critical care medicine personnel. Resuscitation capability depends on common sense, a flexible approach to emergency situations and rapid, almost reflex actions, employed in a titrated fashion, with a sound mix of science and art. It calls as well for appreciation of time factors (speed of action), attention to technical details, and evaluation of outcome. These can be acquired only with experience and objective evaluation of one's own performance. Knowledge gained through reading does not guarantee the ability to resuscitate effectively. There is no substitute for first-hand practical experience. Emergency resuscitation (CPCR) and long-term resuscitation (intensive therapy) are «treatment by titration», in contradistinction to the «treatment by prescription» of standard medical practice.

Those involved in resuscitation must be able to function as team members and/or team leaders. Patient outcome after resuscitation attempts depends in part on the correct deployment of the steps described in this manual, throughout all components of the emergency and critical care medicine delivery system, prehospital and intrahospital. Too often the outcome is determined by the weakest step or component. Thus, physicians in general and anesthesiologists in particular must concern themselves with the educational and organizational aspects of resuscitation services within their hospital and community. Nurses and paramedics are increasingly becoming co-leaders of pre-hospital resuscitation services and CPR teaching programs.

With worldwide instant communication now possible, the World Federation of Societies of Anesthesiologists, World Health Organization, Club of Mainz for Emergency and Disaster Medicine worldwide, and other international professional organizations concerned with resuscitation, should or will jointly review existing knowledge and foster adoption and periodic ungrading of international guidelines concerning «what, whom and how» to teach.

CPCR can make an impact not only in industrialized but also in *developing countries*. Based on needs and present cost-effectiveness, the order of priority for new or expanding programs, particularly in third world countries, should be as follows: (1) life supporting first aid and basic life support training for as many lay persons as possible, and for all health care personnel, particularly those staffing ambulances, emergency and first aid stations and hospitals; this is relatively inexpensive. (2) Pre-hospital advanced life support by mobile ICU ambulances and fixed life support units, as part of a community-wide emergency medical services system, and intra-hospital advanced life support; this is expensive but can be highly cost-effective. (3) Intra-hospital prolonged life support (intensive therapy) for multiple organ failure; this is expensive and often has low cost-effectiveness. Emergency resuscitation is inexpensive and can often eliminate the need for subsequent, expensive intensive care. Thus, in poor countries, upgrading of ambulance services and emergency departments should receive priority over establishing hospital ICUs with electronic monitors and computers. In regions where overwhelming lethal problems like *starvation* and *epidemics* must receive highest priority, even emergency resuscitation has to receive lower priority.

However, what we have learned from emergency care education and organization may in part be effective for improving health care in general in poor regions (Caroline).

Resuscitation practiced with reason and compassion should aim at restoring not only respiratory and circulatory functions, but human mentation as well. The brain must be the target organ of resuscitation. Modern resuscitation has made a medical impact by saving individuals whose lives otherwise would have been cut short before «their time to die has come». However, by asserting that each human life is intrinsically valuable, resuscitation also has a *philosophic impact,* which is at least as important as its potential impact on public health. In a world where human life is often regarded as cheap, resuscitation can be a positive force in the evolution of mankind.

ABBREVIATIONS, DEFINITIONS, NORMAL VALUES

acidemia	Arterial pH less than 7.35
acidosis	Reduced pH (tissues)
alkalemia	Arterial pH greater than 7.45
alkalosis	Increased pH (tissues)
anoxia	No oxygen
apnea	No breathing movements
ARDS	Adult respiratory distress syndrome. Shock lung. Progressive pulmonary consolidation.
arterial oxygen transport ($\overset{\circ}{C}aO_2$)	Cardiac output ($\overset{\circ}{Q}_T$) (resting adult value about 5 liters/min.) times arterial oxygen content (CaO_2) (20 ml/dl) = 1 liter per min.
asphyxia	Hypoxemia plus hypercarbia (due to airway obstr. or apnea)
asystole	Cessation of circulation with heart in standstill (not pumping); electric asystole (EKG isoelectric); mechanical asystole (pulselessness with or without EKG complexes. See EMD).
A-V block	Atrioventricular block (heart)
BD	Blood base deficit. (Negative of BE, base excess). Normal value 0 ± 3 mEq/liter
BP (or AP)	Barometric pressure (Atmospheric pressure) 760 mm Hg at sea level
$^{\circ}\overset{\circ}{C}$	Centigrade (degrees Celsius). See also $^{\circ}F$
CaO_2	Arterial oxygen transport
CaO_2	Arterial oxygen content (20 ml/dl)
cardiac output	$\overset{\circ}{Q}_T$, see arterial oxygen transport
CCM	Critical Care Medicine
CNS	Central Nervous System
CO_2	Carbon dioxide
COP	Colloid osmotic pressure. In plasma 25 torr
CPAP	Continuous Positive Airway Pressure
CPP	Cerebral perfusion pressure, torr; (MAP minus ICP or jugular vein pressure, whichever is higher)
CSF	Cerebrospinal fluid
CVP	Central venous pressure, 3-8 torr
dl	deciliter (100 ml)
ECC	External cardiac (chest) compressions
ECF	Extracellular fluid
ECG(EKG)	Electrocardiogram (-graph)
ED	Emergency Department
EEG	Electroencephalogram (-graph)
EM(EMS)	Emergency Medicine (Emergency Medical Services)
EMD	Electromechanical dissociation, i.e., mechanical asystole with EKG complexes (not VF, VT)
$^{\circ}F$	Degrees Fahrenheit. $^{\circ}F = 32 + 9/5 \ ^{\circ}C$. [$32^{\circ}F = 0^{\circ}C$; $222^{\circ}F = 100^{\circ}C$]

FIO_2	Fraction (concentration) of inhaled oxygen. FIO_2 of air = 0.21 or 21%.
FRC	Functional residual capacity (resting lung volume)
$[H]^+$	Hydrogen ion concentration. See pH
Hb	Hemoglobin content. 13-15 grams/dl
Hct	Hematocrit. 35-45%
$[HCO_3]$	bicarbonate ion concentration. Art. $[HCO_3]$ = 24 mEq/l (calculated from $PaCO_2$ and pHa).
Hypercarbia	$PaCO_2$ greater than 45 torr = Hypercapnia. Due to hypoventilation.
Hypocarbia	$PaCO_2$ less than 35 torr = Hypocapnia. Due to hyperventilation.
Hypoxemia	Arterial PO_2 less than 75 torr
Hypoxia	Reduced oxygen (tissues)
ICP	Intracranial pressure. Less than 15 torr
ICU	Intensive Care Unit
IMV	Intermittent mandatory ventilation (spontaneous breathing plus controlled ventilation)
IPPB	Intermittent positive pressure (assisted) breathing
IPPV	Intermittent positive pressure (controlled) ventilation
IV	Intravenous
Joules	Value of electric energy, = Watt-seconds
kPa	kilo-Pascal (pressure, tension). 1 kPa = 7.5 torr. 5.3 kPa = 40 torr (normal $PaCO_2$). 13.3 kPa = 100 torr (normal PaO_2)
MAP	Mean arterial pressure. 90 ± 10 torr.
MAST	Military (medical) anti-shock trousers. Pressure suit.
mmHg	millimeters of mercury (pressure, tension). 1 mmHg = 1 torr = 0.133 kPa
mEq	milliequivalents
mOsm	milliosmols
$NaHCO_3$	Sodium bicarbonate. See HCO_3^-.
O_2	Oxygen (21% in air)
Oxygen consumption	$\dot{V}O_2$ (resting adult value about 300 ml/70 kg per min)
Pa	Pascal see kPa
$PaCO_2$	Arterial CO_2 tension (pressure). 35-45 torr
PaO_2	Arterial O_2 tension (pressure). With FIO_2 = 21%, PaO_2 = 75-100 torr. With FIO_2 = 100%, PaO_2 = 500-600 torr (less indicates increased shunting).
PA-aO_2	Alveolar-arterial PO_2 difference. Changes (with FIO_2 50 or 100%) reflect changes in $\dot{Q}_S/\dot{Q}_T$. See PaO_2.
PAP	Pulmonary artery pressure. 25/10 torr. Mean PAP 15 (14-17) torr
PAWP	Pulmonary artery wedge pressure. 10 (6-12) torr
PEEP	Positive end-expiratory pressure
pHa	Negative logarithm of hydrogen ion concentration in art. blood. 7.35-7.45.
PNPV	Positive-negative pressure (controlled) ventilation
psi	Pounds per square inch

PVC	Premature ventricular contraction (ventricular extrasystole)
$\overset{\circ}{Q}_T$	Cardiac output (total blood flow). See arterial oxygen transport.
$\overset{\circ}{Q}_S/\overset{\circ}{Q}_T$	Pulmonary shunt (fraction of cardiac output shunted through nonventilated alveoli) $< 10\%$. See $PA\text{-}aO_2$.
SB	Spontaneous breathing
torr	Unit of pressure (tension). Named for Torricelli. 1 torr $= 1$ mmHg $= 0.133$ kPa
$\overset{\circ}{V}O_2$	Oxygen consumption
VF	Ventricular fibrillation
VT	Ventricular tachycardia
W-sec	Watts times seconds $=$ Joules (J) $=$ energy $=$ power x time
Watt	Volts times Amperes $=$ power
WFSA	World Federation of Societies of Anesthesiologists

BIBLIOGRAPHY

Abouleish E: Pain Control in Obstetrics. Philadelphia, Lippincott Publ., 1978.

Abramson NS, Meisel A, Safar P: Resuscitation research and human rights. J Am Med Assoc, submitted 1981.

Ahnefeld FW, Bergmann H, Burric Z, Dick W, Halmagy IM, Rügheimer E: Notfallmedizin. Klinische Anaesthesiologie und Intensive Therapie. Vol 10. Heidelberg, Springer-Verlag, 1975.

Alderman EL: Analgesics in the acute phase of myocardial infarction. J Am Med Assoc 220:1646, 1974.

Alifimoff JK, Safar P, Bircher N, et al: Cardiac resuscitability and cerebral recovery after closed-chest, MAST augmented and open-chest CPR. Anesthesiology 53:S151; 53:S147, 1980.

Ambersen W R, Flecksner J, Steggerda FR, et al: On use of Ringer-Locke solutions containing hemoglobin as substitute for normal blood in mammals. J Cell Compar Physiol 5:359, 1934.

American Heart Association and National Research Council: Standards and guidelines for cardiopulmonary resuscitation and emergency cardiac care. J Am Med Assoc 198:372, 1966; 227:833, 1974; 244:453, 1980.

American EEG Society: Cerebral death and the EEG. JAMA 209:1505, 1969.

American Society of Anesthesiologists Committee on Acute Medicine (Safar P, Chairman): Community-wide emergency medical services. J Am Med Assoc 204:595, 1968.

Ames A III, Wright RL, Kowada M: Cerebral ischemia. II. The no-reflow phenomenon. Am J Pathol 52:437, 1968.

Apgar V: A proposal for a new method of evaluation of the newborn infant. Anesth Analg 32:260, 1953.

Asmussen E, Hahn-Petersen A, Rosendal T: Air passage through the hypopharynx in unconscious patients in the prone position. Acta Anaesth Scand 3:123, 1959.

Astrup P: In Mellemgaard K, Astrup P: The quantitative determination of surplus amounts of acid or base in the human body. Scand J Clin Lab Invest 12:187, 1960.

Babbs CF, Redding JF, Safar P, Tacker WA, eds: Cardiopulmonary Resuscitation. Third Purdue Conference Proceedings. (a) Crit Care Med 8:117, 1980. (b) Med Instrumentation 14:1, 1980.

Babbs CF, Bircher N, Burkett DE, et al: Effect of thoracic venting on arterial pressure and flow during external CPR in animals. Am Heart J submitted.

Baskett P J, Diamond A W, Cochrane D F: Urban mobile resuscitation: training and service. Brit J Anaest 48:377, 1976.

Bates D, Caronna TJ, Cartlidge NEF, et al: A prospective study of non-traumatic coma: methods and results in 310 patients. Annals of Neurology 2:211, 1977.

Beck CS, Pritchard H, Feil SH: Ventricular fibrillation of long duration abolished by electric shock. J Am Med Assoc 135:985, 1947.

Beck CF, Leighninger DS: Death after a clean bill of health. J Am Med Assoc 174:133, 1960.

Becker D: In Vries JK, Becker DPR, Young HF: A subarachnoid screw for monitoring intracranial pressure. J Neurosurg 39:416, 1973.

Beecher H: Harvard Medical School Ad Hoc Committee to examine the definition of brain death: A definition of irreversible coma. J Am Med Assoc 205:337, 1968.

Benson DM, Esposito G, Dorsch J, et al: Mobile intensive care by «unemployable» blacks trained as emergency medical technicians (EMTs) in 1967−69. J Trauma 12:408, 1971.

Benson DM, Stewart C: Inadequacy of pre-hospital emergency care. Crit Care Med 1:130, 1973.

Benson DM, Weigel J: Advanced life support by volunteer fire department ambulance personnel. J Am Coll Emerg Physicians 4:119, 1975.

Berkebile P, Benson D, Ersoz C, et al: Public Education in Heart-Lung Resuscitation. Evaluation of three self-training methods in teenagers. (a) Crit Care Med 1:115, 1973. (b) Proc National Conf on CPR 1973, Dallas, Am Heart Assoc, 1975. (c) Crit Care Med 4:134, 1976.

Bircher NG, Safar P, Stewart R: A comparison of standard, MAST-augmented, and open-chest CPR in dogs. Crit Care Med 8:147, 1980.

Bircher N, Safar P: Comparison of standard and «new» closed-chest CPR and open-chest CPR in dogs. Crit Care Med, May 1981, in press.

Bishop R, Weisfeldt ML: Sodium bicarbonate during cardiac arrest. Effect of arterial pH, PCO_2 and osmolality. J Am Med Assoc 235:506, 1976.

Blalock A: Principles of Surgical Care, Shock and Other Problems. St. Louis, Mosby Publ, 1940.

Bleyaert AL, Nemoto EM, Safar P, et al.: Thiopental amelioration of brain damage after global ischemia in monkeys. (a) Physiologist 18:145, 1975. (b) Acta Neurol Scand 56 (Suppl. 64):144, 1977. (c) Anesthesiology 49:390, 1978.

Bleyaert AL, Sands PA, Safar P, et al.: Augmentation of post-ischemic brain damage by severe intermittent hypertension. Crit Care Med 8:41, 1980.

Bleyaert A, Safar P, Nemoto E, et al.: Effect of post-circulatory-arrest life-support on neurological recovery in monkeys. Crit Care Med 8:153, 1980.

Boehm R: Über Wiederbelebung nach Vergiftungen und Asphyxie. Arch Exp. Pathol Pharmakol 8:68, 1878.

Breivik H, Safar P, Sands P, et al.: Clinical feasibility trials of barbiturate therapy after cardiac arrest. Crit Care Med 6:227, 1978.

Breivik H, Ulvik NM, Blikra G, et al. Life-supporting first aid self-training. Crit Care Med 8:659, 1980.

Brinkmeyer S, Safar P, Motoyama E, et al: Superiority of colloid over electrolyte solution for fluid resuscitation. Crit Care Med, May 1981 in press.

Brophy T: Resuscitation in the Electrical Industry. Brisbane, Electricity Commission of Queensland, 1978.

Brown DC, Lewis AJ, Criley JM: Asystole and its treatment: the possible role of the parasympathetic nervous system in cardiac arrest. J Am Coll Em Phys 8:448, 1979.

Carden NI, Steinhaus JE: Lidocaine resuscitation from ventricular fibrillation. Circ Res 4:640, 1956.

Caroline NL: Medical Care in the Streets. J Am Med Assoc 237:43, 1977.

Caroline NL: Emergency Care in the Streets. Boston, Little Brown Publ, 1979.

Caroline NL: Ambulance calls. Review Problems in Emergency Care. Boston, Little Brown Publ, 1980.

Carroll R, Hedden M, Safar P: Intratracheal cuffs: performance characteristics. Anesthesiology 31:275, 1969.

Carveth SW, Burnap TK, Bechtel J, et al.: Training in advanced cardiac life support. J Am Med Assoc 235:2311, 1976.

Chaillou A: La serum-therapie et le tubage du larynx dans les croups diphteriques. Paris, 1895.

Chandra N, Rudikoff MT, Weisfeldt ML: Simultaneous chest compression and ventilation at high airway pressure during cardiopulmonary resuscitation. Lancet 1:175, 1980.

Cobb LA: In — (a) Cobb LA, Werner JA, Trobaugh GB: Sudden cardiac death. A decade's experience with out of hospital resuscitation. Modern concepts of cardiovasc dis (Am Heart Assoc) 49/6,7:1,37, 1980. (b) Eisenberg MS, et al: Treatment of out of hospital cardiac arrest with rapid defibrillation by emergency medical technicians. New Engl J Med 302:1379, 1980.

Collinsworth KA, Kalman SM, Harrison DC: The clinical pharmacology of lidocaine as an anti-arrhythmic drug. Circ 40:1217, 1974.

Comroe JH, Dripps RD, Dumke PR, et al: Oxygen toxicity. J Am Med Assoc 128:710, 1945.

Cowley R A, Trump B F (eds.): Pathophysiology of Shock, Anoxia, and Ischemia. Williams and Wilkins, Baltimore, 1981.

Crampton RS, Aldrich RF, Stillerman R: Prehospital CPR in acute myocardial infarction. N Engl J Med 26:132, 1972.

Crile GW: Reported in Keen WW: A case of total laryngectomy (unsuccessful) and a case of an abdominal hysterectomy (successful), in both of which massage of the heart for chloroform collapse was employed, with notes of 25 other cases of cardiac massage. Ther Gaz 28:217, 1904.

Crile G, Dolley DH: An experimental research into the resuscitation of dogs killed by anesthetics and asphyxia. J Exp Med 8:713, 1906.

Criley JM, Blaufuss AH, Kissel GL, et al.: Cough-induced cardiac compression: self-administered form of cardiopulmonary resuscitation. (a) J Am Med Assoc 36:1246, 1976. (b) Crit Care Med 8:141, 1980. (c) Crit Care Med, May 1981 in press.

Criley JM, Niemann JT, Rosborough JP: The heart is a conduit in CPR. Crit Care Med, May 1981 in press.

Dawidson I, Haglind E, Gelin LE: Hemodilution and oxygen transport to tissue in shock. Acta Chir Scand Suppl 489:245, 1979. See also Dawidson I: Hemodilution, oxygen consumption, and recovery from shock:, Univ Göteborg Publ, 1980 (Thesis).

DelGuercio LRM, Feins NR, Cohn JD, et al: A comparison of blood flow during external and internal cardiac massage in man. Circulation 30:63, 1964; 31:1, 1965.

Dembo EH: Calcium in advanced life support. Crit Care Med, May 1981 in press.

Detre K, Abramson N, Safar P, et al: Collaborative randomized clinical study cardiopulmonary-cerebral resuscitation. Crit Care Med, May 1981 in press.

Deming M: Unpublished experiences on pediatric endotracheal anesthesia. See (a) Dripps R, et al: Introduction to Anesthesia. Philadelphia, Saunders Publ, 1957-1980. (b) Eckenhoff JE: Anesthesiology 12:401, 1951.

Don Micheal TA, Lambert EH, Mehran A: Mouth-to-lung airway for cardiac resuscitation. Lancet 2:1329, 1968.

Dortmann C, Droh R, Frey R: Der Mainzer Notarztwagen. Der Anaesthesist 19:212, 1970.

Dripps RD, et al.: Cardiac resuscitation. Ann Surg 127:592, 1948.

Dripps RD, Eckenhoff JE, Vandam LR: Introduction to Anesthesia. Philadelphia, Saunders Publ, 1957-80.

Elam JO, Brown ES, Elder JD, Jr: Artificial respiration by mouth-to-mask method. A study of the respiratory gas exchange of paralyzed patients ventilated by operator's expired air. N Engl J Med 250:749, 1954.

Elam JO, Greene DG, Brown ES, et al: Oxygen and carbon dioxide exchange and energy cost of expired air resuscitation. J Am Med Assoc 167:328, 1958.

Elam JO, Greene DG: Mission accomplished: successful mouth-to-mouth resuscitation. Anesth Analg 40:440, 578, 672, 1961.

Elam JO, ViaReque E, Rattenborg CC: Esophageal electrocardiography and low energy ventricular defibrillation. In Safar P (ed) Advances in CPR. New York, Springer Verlag, 1975.

Engstrom CG: A clinical application of prolonged controlled ventilation. Acta Anaesth Scand, Suppl 13, 1963.

Esmarch JF: The Surgeons Handbook on the Treatment of Wounded in War. New York, Schmidt Publ, 1878, p. 113.

Esposito G, Safar P, Medsger A, Nesbitt J: Life supporting first aid (LSFA) self-training for the lay public. Anesthesiology 53/3:S375, 1980. And Crit Care Med, May 1981 in press.

Fink BR: The etiology and treatment of laryngeal spasm. Anesthesiology 17:569, 1956.

Frey R, Eyrich K, Lutz H, Peter K, Weis K H: Infusionstherapie. Aesopus Verlag, Munich, 1974.

Frey R, Nagel E, Safar P: Mobile intensive care units. Advanced emergency care delivery systems. Symposium Mainz 1973. Anesthesiology and Resuscitation Vol 95. Heidelberg, Springer Verlag, 1976.

Frey R: The Club of Mainz for improved worldwide emergency and critical care medicine systems and disaster preparedness. Crit Care Med 6:389, 1978.

Frey R, Safar P (editors): Disaster Medicine. Internat Congress (Mainz 1977) issues Vol. I, 1979; Vol. II, 1980. Heidelberg, Springer Verlag.

Fryer R: Personal communication 1977 (Pittsburgh).

Gelin LE: (a) Studies in anemia of injury. Acta Anaes Scand Suppl. 210, 1956. (b) Reaction of the body as a whole to injury. J Trauma 10:932, 1970.

Geyer R P, Monroe R G, Taylor K: Survival of rats having red cells totally replaced with emulsified fluorocarbon. N Engl J Med 289:1077, 1973.

Gillespie NA: Endotracheal Anesthesia. Madison, University of Wisconsin Press, 1950.

Gisvold SE, Safar P, Alexander H, et al: Cardiovascular tolerance of thiopental anesthesia for brain resuscitation in monkeys. CBF Symposium, St. Louis 1981. J Cerebral Blood Flow and Metabol, 1981 in press.

Gisvold SE, Safar P, Bleyaert A, et al: No amelioration of post-anoxic brain damage by immobilization and controlled ventilation in monkeys. Preliminary results. CBF Symposium, St. Louis 1981. J. Cerebral Blood Flow and Metabol, 1981 in press.

Goldberg LI: Dopamine — clinical use of an endogenous catecholamine. N Engl J Med 291:707, 1974.

Goldstein A, Wells BA, Keats AS: Increased tolerance to cerebral anoxia by pentobarbital. Arch Intern Pharmacodynamie et de Therapie 161:138, 1966.

Gordon AS, Sadove MS, Raymon F, et al: Critical survey of manual artificial respiration for children and adults. J Am Med Assoc 147:1444, 1951.

Gordon AS, Frye CW, Gittelson L, et al: Mouth-to-mouth versus manual artificial respiration for children and adults. J Am Med Assoc 167:320, 1958.

Gordon AS, Belton MK, Ridolpho PF: Emergency management of foreign body airway obstruction. Comparison of artificial cough techniques, manual extraction maneuvers, and simple mechanical devices. In Safar P (ed) Advances in CPR. New York, Springer Verlag, 1977. p. 39.

Grace WJ, Kennedy RJ, Nolte CT: Blind defibrillation. Am J Cardiol 34:115, 1974.

Greenbaum DM, Millen JE, Eross B, et al: Continuous positive airway pressure without tracheal intubation in spontaneously breathing patients. Chest 69:615, 1976.

Greenbaum DM: Secondary cardiac dysrhythmias. Heart & Lung 6:308, 1977.

Gregory GA: Resuscitation of the newborn. Anesthesiology 43:225, 1975.

Grenvik A, Powner DJ, Snyder JV, et al: Cessation of therapy in terminal illness and brain death. Crit Care Med 6:284, 1978.

Grenvik A (ed.): Brain failure and resuscitation. Clinics in Crit Care Med. Harlow, Churchill-Livingston Publ., 1981.

Guildner CW: Resuscitation — opening the airway. J Am Coll Em Phys 5:588, 1976.

Guildner CW, Williams D, Subitch T: Emergency management for airway obstruction by foreign material. In Safar P (ed) Advances in CPR. New York, Springer Verlag, 1977. pg 51.

Gurvich NL, Yuniev SG: Restoration of a regular rhythm in the mammalian fibrillating heart. Am Rev Sov Med 3:236, 1946.

Gurvitch A M: Determination of the depth and reversibility of postanoxic coma in animals. Resuscitation 3:1, 1974.

Harris LC, Kirimli B, Safar P: Augmentation of artificial circulation during cardiopulmonary resuscitation. Anesthesiology 28:730, 1967.

Harris LC, Kirimli B, Safar P: Ventilation-cardiac compression rates and ratios in cardiopulmonary resuscitation. Anesthesiology 28:806, 1967.

Haugen RK: The cafe coronary. Sudden death in restaurants. J Am Med Assoc 186:142, 1963.

Hedden M, Ersoz CJ, Donnelly WH, et al: Laryngotracheal damage after prolonged use of orotracheal tubes in adults. J Am Med Assoc 207:703, 1969.

Heiberg J: A new expedient in administering chloroform. Medical Times and Gazette, January 10, 1874.

Heimlich HJ: A life-saving maneuver to prevent food choking. J Am Med Assoc 234:398, 1975.

Hingson RA: Western Reserve anesthesia machine, oxygen inhalator and resuscitator. J Am Med Assoc 167:1077, 1958.

Hoff JT: Resuscitation in focal brain ischemia. Crit Care Med 6:245, 1978.

Holmdahl MH: Respiratory care unit. Anesthesiology 23:559, 1962.

Hooker DR, Kouwenhoven WB, Langworthy OR: Effect of alternating electrical currents on the heart. Am J Physiol 103:444, 1933.

Hossli G: Die Behandlung des Bewusstlosen durch den praktischen Arzt. Z Aerztl Fortbild 51:955, 1962.

Hossmann KA, Kleihues P: Reversibility of ischemic brain damage. Arch Neurol 29:375, 1973.

Ibsen B: From anaesthesia to anaesthesiology. Acta Anaes Scand. 19:suppl. 61, 1975.

Ikada S, Yanai N, Ischikawa S: Flexible bronchofiber scope. Keio J Med 17:2, 1968.

Jacobs HB: Emergency percutaneous transtracheal catheter and ventilator. J Trauma 12:50, 1972.

Jacoby JJ, Hamelberg W, Ziegler CH, et al: Transtracheal resuscitation. J Am Med Assoc 162:625, 1956.

Jennett B, Bond M: Assessment of outcome after severe brain damage: a practical scale. Lancet, 1:480, 1975.

Jude JR, Kouwenhoven WB, Knickerbocker GG: Cardiac arrest: report of application of external cardiac massage on 118 patients. J Am Med Assoc 178:1063, 1961.

Jurkiewicz J: The effect of haemodilution on experimental brain edema. Europ J Intensive Care Med 3:167, 1977.

Kampschulte S, Marcy J, Safar P: Simplified physiologic management of status asthmaticus in children. Crit Care Med 1:69, 1973.

Kantrowitz A, Tjønneland S, Freed PS, et al: Initial clinical experience with intraaortic balloon pumping in cardiogenic shock. J Am Med Assoc 203:113, 1968.

Kaplan BC, Civetta JM, Nagel EL, et al: The Military Anti-Shock Trouser in civilian pre-hospital emergency care. J Trauma 13:843, 1973.

Kirby, RR, Robison EJ, Schultz J: A new pediatric volume ventilator. Anesth Analg 50:533, 1971.

Kirimli B, Harris LC, Safar P: Drugs in cardiopulmonary resuscitation. Acta Anaesth Scand (Suppl) 23:255, 1966.

Kirimli B, Kampschulte S, Safar P: Cardiac arrest from exsanguination in dogs. Evaluation of resuscitation methods. Acta Anaesth Scand (Suppl) 39:183, 1968.

Kitterman JA, Phibbs RH, Tooley WH: Catheterization of umbilical vessels in newborn infants. Pediatr Clin North Am 17:895, 1970.

Klain M, Smith RB: High frequency percutaneous transtracheal jet ventilation. Crit Care Med 5:280, 1977.

Klain M, Keszler H, Brader E: High frequency jet ventilation in CPR. Crit Care Med, May 1981 in press.

Koch-Weser J: Drug therapy: Bretylium. N Engl J Med 300:473, 1979.

Kouwenhoven WB, Milner WR: Treatment of ventricular fibrillation using a capacitor discharge. J Appl Physiol 7:253, 1954.

Kouwenhoven WB, Jude JR, Knickerbocker GG: Closed-chest cardiac massage. J Am Med Assoc 173:1064, 1960.

Kucher R, Steinbereithner K: Intensive Therapie. Stuttgart, Thieme Publ 1972, 1980.

Kuhn F: Die perorale Intubation. Berlin, S. Karger Publ, 1911.

Laborit H, Huguenard P: Practice of Hibernation Therapy in Surgery and Medicine (French). Masson, Paris, 1954.

Lane I (ed): Reamimacao. Rio de Janeiro, Guanabara Koogan Publ., 1981, (in Portuguese).

Lawin P: Praxis der Intensivbehandlung. Stuttgart, Thieme Publ. 1975.

Ledingham IM (ed): Clinics in Critical Care Medicine Series. London, Churchill Livingstone Publ, 1980.

Leighninger DS: Contributions of Claude Beck. In Safar P (ed) Advances in CPR. New York, Springer Verlag, 1977. Ch. 38, p. 259.

Lind B: Teaching mouth-to-mouth resuscitation in primary schools. Acta Anesth Scand (Suppl) 9:63, 1961.

Lind B, Stovner J: Mouth-to-mouth resuscitation in Norway. J Am Med Assoc 185:933, 1963.

Lind B, Snyder J, Safar P: Total brain ischemia in dogs: cerebral physiological and metabolic changes after 15 minutes of circulatory arrest. Resuscitation 4:97, 1975.

Lindholm CR: Prolonged endotracheal intubation. Acta Anaesth Scand (Suppl) 33, 1969.

Lown B: Comparison of AC and DC electroshock across the closed chest. Amer J Cardiol 10:223, 1962.

Lund I, Lind B (eds): International Symposium on Emergency Resuscitation, Oslo, Norway, 1967. Acta Anesth Scand (suppl) 29, 1968. (See also Poulsen, 1961).

Lund I, Skulberg A: Cardiopulmonary resuscitation by lay people. Lancet 2:702, 1976.

Lust P: Continuum of physician leadership from the scene via the emergency department to the ICU. Disaster Medicine, Vol. IV. Heidelberg, Springer Verlag, 1982 in press.

Maass: Die Methode der Wiederbelebung bei Herztod nach Chloroformeinathmung. Berlin Klin Wochschr 29:265, 1892.

Macintosh RR: A new laryngoscope. Lancet 1:205, 1943.

Macintosh RR: (a) Oxford inflating bellows. Brit Med J 2:202, 1953. (b) A plea for simplicity. Brit Med J 2:1054, 1955.

Magill IW: Endotracheal anesthesia. Amer J Surg 34:450, 1936.

Mattar JA, Weil MH, Shubin H, et al: Cardiac arrest in the critically ill: II. Hyperosmolal states following cardiac arrest. Am J Med 56:162, 1974.

Mayrhofer O: Wann endet das Leben, Wann beginnt der Tod? Österr. Ärztezeitung 19:2089, 1968. See also textbook of Anesthesiology by R. Frey, W. Hugin, O. Mayrhofer (eds), Heidelberg, Springer Verlag, 1971.

MacKenzie GJ, Taylor SH, McDonald AH, et al: Hemodynamic effects of external cardiac compression. Lancet 1:1345, 1964.

Manni C, Magalini S I, Scrascia E (editors). Total Parenteral Alimentation. American Elsevier Publ., New York, 1976.

Messmer K (ed): Hemodilution, A Symposium. Der Anaesthesist 25:123, 1976.

Michenfelder JD, Theye RA: The effects of anesthesia and hypothermia on canine cerebral ATP and lactate during anoxia produced by decapitation. Anesthesiology 33:430, 1970.

Milai AS, Davis G, Safar P: Simplified apparatus for IPPV/aerosol therapy. Anesthesiology 26:362, 1965.

Mirowski M, Reid PR, Mower MM, et al: Termination of malignant ventricular arrhythmias with an implanted automatic defibrillator in human beings. N Eng J Med 303:322, 1980.

Moerch ET, Avery EE, Benson DW: Hyperventilation in the treatment of crushing injuries of the chest. Surg Forum 6:270, 1956.

Modell JH: The Pathophysiology and Treatment of Drowning and Near-Drowning. Springfield IL, Thomas Publ, 1971.

Moossy J, Reinmuth OM (eds.): Cerebral vascular diseases (12th Research Conference). New York, Raven Press, 1980 in press.

Morikawa S, Safar P, DeCarlo J: Influence of head position upon upper airway patency. Anesthesiology 22:265, 1961.

Muendich K, Hoflehner G: Ventilation bronchoscopy. Der Anaesthesist 2:121, 1953.

Mullie A, Lust P, Penninckx J, et al: Monitoring of cerebro-spinal fluid enzyme levels in postischemic encephalopathy after cardiac arrest. Crit Care Med, May 1981 in press.

Mushin WW, Rendell-Baker L, Thompson PW, et al: Automatic ventilation of the lungs. Philadelphia, Davis Publ, 1969.

Nagel EL, Hirschman JC, Nussenfeld SR, et al: Telemetry-medical command in coronary and other mobile emergency care systems. J Am Med Assoc 214: 332, 1970. See also: Liberthson RR, Nagel EL, Hirschman JC, et al: Prehospital ventricular fibrillation. Prognosis and follow-up course. N Engl J Med 291:317, 1974.

Naito R, Yokoyama K: On the perfluorodecalin/phospholipid emulsion as the red cell substitute. In Proceedings of the 10th International Nutrition Symposium on PFC Artificial Blood, p. 55. Kyoto, 1975.

Negovsky VA: Reanimatology — The Science of Resuscitation. In Stephenson HE: Cardiac Arrest and Resuscitation. St. Louis, Mosby Publ, 1974.

Negovsky VA: Current Problems in Reanimatology. Moscow, Mir Publ, 1975.

Nemoto EM: Pathogenesis of cerebral ischemia-anoxia. Crit Care Med 6:203, 1978.

Nemoto EM, Erdman NW, Strong E, et al: Regional brain PO_2 after global ischemia in monkeys: evidence for regional differences in critical perfusion pressures. Stroke 10:44, 1979.

Nilsson E. On treatment of barbiturate poisoning. A modified clinical aspect. Acta Med Scand (suppl) 253, 1951.

Nobel J, et al, In Health Devices (Emergency Care Research Institute, 5200 Butler Pike, Plymouth Meeting, PA 19462 USA): (a) Manually operated resuscitators, 1:13, 1971. (b) Defibrillators, 1:109, 1971; 2:87, 1973; 1:117, 1973. (c) External heart compressors, 2:136, 1973.

Otto CW, Yakaitis RW: Comparison of dopamine, dobutamine, epinephrine and other sympathomimetic amines in CPR. See Purdue Conference (Babbs C), and Wolf Creek Conference #2 (Redding J). Also Crit. Care Med. May 1981 in press.

Palmer RF, Lasseter KC: Sodium nitroprusside. N Engl J Med 292:294, 1975.

Pantridge JF, Geddes JS: A mobile intensive care unit in the management of myocardial infarction. Lancet 2:271, 1967.

Pearson J, Safar P: General anesthesia with minimal equipment. Anesth Analg 40:664, 1961.

Pearson JW, Redding JS: Influence of peripheral vascular tone on cardiac resuscitation. Anesth Analg 44:746, 1965.

Peieska B: Transthoracic and direct defibrillation. Rozhl Chir (CSSR) 26:731, 1957.

Pennington JE, Taylor J, Lown B: Chest thump for reverting ventricular tachycardia. N Engl J Med 283:1192, 1970.

Petty TL, Ashbaugh DG: The adult respiratory distress syndrome. Chest 60:233, 1971.

Plum F (ed): Symposium on Brain Ischemia. Arch Neurol 29:1, 1973.

Pontoppidan H, Geffin B, Lowenstein E: Acute respiratory failure in the adult. Boston, Little Brown Publ, 1973.

Poulsen H (ed): International Symposium on Emergency Resuscitation, Stavanger, Norway, 1960. Acta Anaesth Scand (Suppl) 9, 1961. (See also Lund, 1968).

Prevost JL, Battelli F: On some effects of electrical discharges on the hearts of mammals. Compt Rend Acad Sci (Paris) 129:1267, 1899.

Ravitch M, Lane R, Safar P, et al: Lightning Stroke. Recovery following cardiac massage and prolonged artificial respiration. N Engl J Med 264:36, 1961.

Redding J, Cozine R: A Comparison of open-chest and closed-chest cardiac massage in dogs. Anesthesiology 22:280, 1961.

Redding J, Cozine RA, Voigt GC, et al: Resuscitation from drowning. J Am Med Assoc 178:1136, 1961.

Redding JS, Pearson JW: Evaluation of drugs for cardiac resuscitation. Anesthesiology 24:203, 1963.

Redding JS, Asuncion JS, Pearson JW: Effective routes of drug administration during cardiac arrest. Anesth Analg 46:253, 1967.

Redding JS: Abdominal compression in CPR. Anesthesiology 50:668, 1971.

Redding JS: Precordial thumping during cardiac resuscitation. In Safar P (ed) Advances in CPR. New York, Springer, 1977, p. 87.

Redding JS: The choking controversy. Crit Care Med 8:184, 1980.

Redding JS (ed): Wolf Creek Conference on CPR # 2. Crit Care Med, May 1981 (See also Safar, 1977).

Resnekov L: Calcium antagonist drugs-myocardial preservation and reduced vulnerability to ventricular fibrillation. Crit Care Med, May 1981 in press.

Rosen M, Hillard EK: The use of suction in clinical medicine. Brit J Anaesth 32:486, 1960.

Rosomoff HL, Shulman K, Raynor R, et al: Experimental brain injury and delayed hypothermia. Surg Gynecol Obstet 110:27, 1960.

Royal Colleges of the United Kingdom: Diagnosis of brain death. Brit Med J 2:1187, 1976.

Ruben H: Combination resuscitator and aspirator. Anesthesiology 19:408, 1958.

Ruben H, Knudsen EJ, Carugati G: Gastric inflation in relation to airway pressure. Acta Anaesth Scand 5:107, 1961.

Ruben H, MacNaughton FI: The treatment of food-choking. Practitioner 221:725, 1978.

Rudikoff M T, Maughan W L, Effron M, et al: Mechanisms of blood flow during cardiopulmonary resuscitation. Circulation 61:345, 1980.

Safar P: Mouth-to-mouth airway. Anesthesiology 18:904, 1957.

Safar P, Escarraga L, Elam J: A comparison of the mouth-to-mouth and mouth-to-airway methods of artificial respiration with the chest-pressure arm-lift methods. N Engl J Med 258:671, 1958.

Safar P: Ventilatory efficacy of mouth-to-mouth artificial respiration. Airway obstruction during manual and mouth-to-mouth artificial respiration. J Am Med Assoc 167:335, 1958.

Safar P: Ventilating bronchoscope. Anesthesiology 19:407, 1958.

Safar P, Aguto-Escarraga L, Chang F: A study of upper airway obstruction in the unconscious patient. J Appl Physiol 14:760, 1959.

Safar P, Brown TC, Holtey WH, et al: Ventilation and circulation with closed chest cardiac massage in man. J Am Med Assoc 176:574, 1961.

Safar P, DeKornfeld TJ, Pearson JW, et al: Intensive care unit. Anaesthesia 16:275, 1961.

Safar P, Berman B, Diamond E, et al: Cuffed tracheostomy tube vs. tank respirator for prolonged artificial ventilation. Arch Phys Med Rehabil. 43:487, 1962.

Safar P, Tenicela R: High altitude physiology in relation to anesthesia and inhalation therapy. Anesthesiology 25:515, 1964.

Safar P, Penninckx J: Cricothyroid membrane puncture with special cannula. Anesthesiology 28:943, 1967.

Safar P, Benson DM, Brose RA, et al: Ambulance design and equipment, and emergency medical technicians training. (a) Arch Surg 90:343, 1965. (b) Arch Surg 102:163, 1971. (c) Anesth Analg 51:27, 1972.

Safar P: Pocket mask for emergency artificial ventilation and oxygen inhalation. Crit Care Med 2:273, 1974.

Safar P (ed): Public Health Aspects of Critical Care Medicine and Anesthesiology. Philadelphia, Davis Publ, 1974. Chapters 4, 6 (EMS Organization).

Safar P, Benson DM, Berkebile PE, et al: Teaching and Organizing CPR. In: Safar P (ed), Public Health Aspects of CCM and Anes. Philadelphia, Davis Publ, 1974. Chapter 7, pags. 161-192.

Safar P, Lind B: Triple airway maneuver, artificial ventilation and oxygen inhalation by mouth-to-mask and bag-valve-mask techniques. Proc National Conf on CPR 1973, Dallas, Am Heart Assoc, 1975. p. 49.

Safar P, Scott MA, Ricci E, et al: CPR self-training systems and impact evaluation. Nat Instit Health (USA) Project HR-42965 (1974—77). Disaster Med. New York, Springer Verlag, 1982.

Safar P, Stezoski SW, Nemoto EM: Amelioration of brain damage after 12 minutes cardiac arrest in dogs. Arch Neurol 33:91, 1976.

Safar P, Elam J (eds): Advances in CPR. Wolf Creek Conference on CPR #1, 1975. New York, Springer Verlag, 1977. (See also Redding, 1981).

Safar P, Grenvik A: Organization and physician education in critical care medicine. Anesthesiology 47:82, 1977.

Safar P, Caroline N, et al: Teaching texts on CPR and long-term intensive care life support. Chapters 2-10 in: Schwartz G, et al (eds): Principles and Practice of Emergency Medicine. Philadelphia, Saunders Publ. 1978, 1984.

Safar P (ed): Brain Resuscitation. Special Issue. Crit Care Med 6:199-291, 1978.

Safar P: Pathophysiology and resuscitation of global brain ischemia. (a) Internat Anesth Clinics 17:239-284, 1979. (b) Brain Failure and Resuscitation (Grenvik A, ed). Clinics in Critical Care Medicine. Harlow, Churchill-Livingston Publ, 1981.

Safar P, Abramson N, Detre K, et al: Multi-institutional international randomized clinical study of cardiopulmonary-cerebral resuscitation. Nat Instit Health (USA) Project NS-15295 (1979-83). See Detre, Mullie, Breivik.

Safar P: Amelioration of Postischemic Brain Damage with Barbiturates. Stroke 15:1, 1980.

Sassano J, Eshel G, Safar P, et al: Hyperthermic cardiac arrest in monkeys. Crit Care Med, May 1981 in press.

Schiff M: Über direkte Reizung der Herzoberfläche. Arch Ges Physiol 28:200, 1882.

Schofferman J, Oill P, Lewis AJ: The esophageal obturator airway. A clinical evaluation. Chest 69:67, 1976.

Schwartz AJ, Orkin FK, Ellison N: Anesthesiologists' training and knowledge of basic life support. Anesthesiology 50:191, 1979.

Schwartz G, Safar P, Stone J, et al (eds): Principles and Practice of Emergency Medicine. Philadelphia, Saunders Publ, 1978, 1984.

Secher O, Wilhjelm B: The protective action of anesthetics against hypoxia. Canad Anaesth Soc J 15:423, 1968.

Seeley S: Accidental Death and Disability: The Neglected Disease of Modern Society. Committee on Trauma and Committee on Shock, Division of Medical Sciences. Washington, DC, National Academy of Sciences, National Research Council, 1966.

Sefrna B: Pre-hospital advanced life support experiences in Prague. (Personal communication), 1962.

Sellick BA: Cricoid pressure to control regurgitation of stomach contents during induction of anesthesia. Lancet 2:404, 1961.

Severinghaus J: Blood gas concentrations. Chapter 61, in Handbook of Physiology Vol. II, Section 3, Respiration. Page 1475. Washington, Am Physiol Soc, 1965.

Shapiro HM: Intracranial hypertension. Anesthesiology 43:445, 1975.

Shoemaker WC: Comparison of the relative effectiveness of whole blood transfusions and various types of fluid therapy in resuscitation. Crit Care Med 4:71, 1976.

Shoemaker W, Thompson L, (eds): Critical Care Medicine: State of the Art Vol. I, 1980; Vol. II, 1981. Anaheim, California, Soc Crit Care Med Publ.

Shubin H, Weil MH, Carlson RW, et al: Cardiovascular system failure. In Schwartz G, et al (eds) Principles and Practice of Emergency Medicine. Philadelphia, Saunders Publ., 1978. Chapter 4, p. 104.

Siebke H, Rod T, Breivik H: Survival after 40 minutes submersion without cerebral sequelae. Lancet 1:1275, 1975.

Siggaard-Andersen O: Blood acid base alignment nomogram. Scales for pH, PCO_2, base excess of whole blood of different hemoglobin concentration, plasma bicarbonate and plasma total CO_2. Scand J Clin Lab Invest 15:211, 1963.

Singh NP: Transtracheal jet ventilation as a new technique and experiences with ketamine and propandid in India. In «Anesthesiology» (WFSA Congress Kyoto, 1972) (Miyazaki M, ed). Amsterdam, Excerpta Medica, 1973, pg. 160.

Siesjo BK. Brain Energy Metabolism. New York, John Wiley Publ, 1978.

Sjöstrand U, (ed): Experimental and clinical evaluation of high frequency positive pressure ventilation. Acta Anaes Scand 64:1, 1977.

Smetana J, Racenberg E, Juna S: Resuscitation of the heart; experimental study and clinical experience. Rev Czech Med 7:65, 1961.

Smith AL, Hoff JT, Nielson SL: Barbiturate protection against cerebral infarction. Stroke 5:1, 1974.

Smith J, Penninckx JJ, Kampschulte S, et al: Need for oxygen enrichment in myocardial infarction, shock, and following cardiac arrest. Acta Anaesth Scand (Suppl) 29:127, 1968.

Smith RB, Schaer WB, Pfaeffle H: Percutaneous transtracheal ventilation for anesthesia and resuscitaion: a review and report of complications. Canad Anaesth Soc J 22:607, 1975.

Snyder JV, Nemoto EM, Carroll RG, et al: Global ischemia in dogs: intracranial pressures, brain blood flow and metabolism. Stroke 6:21, 1975.

Snyder JV, Powner DJ, Grenvik A: Neurologic intensive care. In Cottrell JE (ed), Anesthesia and Neurosurgery. St. Louis, Mosby Publ, 1973.

Spoerel WE, Narayanan PS, Singh NP: Transtracheal ventilation. Br J Anaesth 43:932, 1971.

Steen P A, Michenfelder J D, Milde J H: Incomplete versus complete cerebral ischemia: Improved outcome with a minimal blood flow. Ann Neurol 6:389, 1979.

Stephenson HE: Cardiac Arrest and Resuscitation. St. Louis, Mosby Publ. 1974.

Stept WJ, Safar P: Rapid induction/intubation for prevention of gastric content aspiration. Anesth Analg 49:633, 1970.

Stewart JS: Management of cardiac arrest with special reference to metabolic acidosis. Br. Med J 1:476, 1964.

Stewart RV: CPR in prehospital care. Topics in Emerg Med 1:1, 1979. Also personal communication.

Suter PM, Fairley, HB, Isenberg MD: The optimum end-expiratory airway pressure in patients with acute pulmonary failure. N Engl J Med 292:284, 1975.

Swan HJC, Ganz W, Forrester J, et al: Catheterization of the heart in man with use of a flow-directed balloon-tipped catheter. N Engl J Med 283:447, 1970.

Tacker WA Jr, Wey GA: Emergency defibrillation dose: Recommendations and rationale. Circulation 60:223, 1979.

Takaori M, Safar P: Treatment of massive hemorrhage with colloid and crystalloid solutions. J Am Med Assoc 199:297, 1967.

Takaori M, Safar P: Critical point in progressive hemodilution with hydroxyethyl starch. Kawasaki Med. J. 2:211, 1976.

Teasdale G, Jennett B: Assessment of coma and impaired consciousness. A practical scale. Lancet 2:81, 1974.

Thompson W L: Rational use of albumin and plasma substitutes. Johns Hopkins Med J 136:220, 1975.

Torpey DJ: Resuscitation and Anesthetic Management of Casualties. J Am Med Assoc 202:955, 1967.

Tossach WA: A man dead in appearance recovered by distending the lungs with air. In Medical Essays and Observations. London, Caldell and Balfour, 108-111, 1771.

Trubuhovich RV (ed.): Management of acute intracranial disasters. Internat Anesth Clinics 17/2-3, 1979.

Tuttle RR, Mills J: Dobutamine: Development of a new catecholamine to selectively increase cardiac contractility. Circ Res 36:185, 1975.

Vesalius A: De corporis humani fabrica. Libri Septem, 1543.

Valentine PA, Frew JL, Mashford ML, et al: Lidocaine in the prevention of sudden death in the prehospital phase of acute infarction. N Engl J Med 291:1327, 1974.

Walt AJ, Wilson RF: Management of trauma, pitfalls in practice. Philadelphia, Lea Febiger Publ, 1975.

Waters RM, Rovenstein EA, Guedel AE: Endotracheal anesthesia and its historical development. Anesthesiology 12:196, 1933.

Weil MH, Shubin H: The «VIP» approach to the bedside management of shock. J Am Med Assoc. 207:337, 1969.

Weil MH, Shubin H (eds): Critical Care Medicine, Current Principles and Practice. Hagerstown, Harper & Rowe Publ., 1976.

Weil MH, Henning RJ. New concepts in the diagnosis and fluid treatment of circulatory shock. Anesth. Analg 58:124, 1979.

Weisfeldt ML, Chandra N, Tsitlik J: Increased intrathoracic pressure — not direct heart compression — causes the rise in intrathoracic vascular pressures during CPR in dogs and pigs. Crit Care Med, May 1981. (See also Chandra, Rudikoff, Bircher, Criley).

White B C, Petinga T J, Hoehner P J, et al: Incidence, etiology, and outcome of pulseless idioventricular rhythm treated with dexamethasone during advanced CPR. J Amer Coll Emerg Phys 8:188, 1979.

Wiggers CJ: The physiological bases for cardiac resuscitation from ventricular fibrillation. Method for serial defibrillation. Am Heart J 20:413, 1940.

Wilder RJ, Weir D, Rush BF, et al: Methods of coordinating ventilation and closed-chest cardiac massage in the dog. Surgery 53:186, 1963.

Wilder RJ, Jude JR, Kouwenhoven WB: Cardiopulmonary resuscitation by trained ambulance personnel. J Am Med Assoc 190:531, 1964.

Winchell SW, Safar P: Teaching and testing lay and paramedical personnel in cardio-pulmonary resuscitation. Anes Analg 45:441, 1966.

Winter P, Smith G, Miller JN: The toxicity of oxygen. A symposium review. Anesthesiology 37:210, 1972. See also Miller JN, Winter PM: Clinical manifestations of pulmonary oxygen toxicity. Boston, Little Brown Publ, 1979.

Yakaitis RW, Redding JS: Precordial thumping during cardiac resuscitation. Crit Care Med 1:22, 1973.

Yatsu FM, Diamond I, Graziana C, et al: Experimental brain ischemia; protection from irreversible damage with a rapid-acting barbiturate (methohexital). Stroke, 3:726, 1972.

Zindler M, Dudziak R, Pulver KG: Artificial hypothermia (in German) Chapter C/12/c, p. 353. In Anesthesiologie und Wiederbelebung, Frey R, et al (eds), Heidelberg, Springer Verlag, 1971.

Zipes EP, Troup EJ: New anti-arrhythmic agents: Amiodarone, aprindine, disopyramide, ethmozin, mexiletine, tocainide, verapamil. Amer J Cardiol 41:1005, 1978.

Zoll PM, Linenthal AJ, Gibson W: Termination of ventricular fibrillation in man by externally applied electric countershock. N Engl J Med 254:727, 1956.

Zoll PM, Linenthal AJ, Norman LR: Treatment of Unexpected cardiac arrest by external stimulation of the heart. N Engl J Med 254:541, 1956.

Zorab J, Baskett P: Immediate care. Philadelphia, Saunders Publ. 1977.

INDEX
(pages)

For authors, see text and bibliography.
For abbreviations, see glossary, then index.

Abbreviations 217
ABC sequence 87
abdominal restraint 87
abdominal thrusts 26, 27, 28, 164
AC defibrillation 131, 132, 134
ACD blood preservation 120
acid base status nomogram 72, 109
acidemia, acidosis 91, 108, 165, 178
Adams-Stokes syndrome 170
administrator 204
adrenaline (epinephrine) 53, 94, 102
adult respiratory distress syndrome (ARDS) 69, 138
advanced life support 11, 15, 92, 185, 193, 195, 203, 204, 211, 212
aerosol-oxygen 53, 72
agonal state 174
aircraft 209, 210
airway control 11, 16, 51, 139, 191
airway obstruction 16, 31, 76, 193
airway pressure 57, 73, 166
albumin 117, 119, 139, 167
algorithm 196
aligned position 91, 93
alimentation 139, 141
alkalemia 108
Allen's test 100
alpha receptors 103
altitude 75
alveolar dysfunction 76
alveolar rupture 53
alveolar ventilation 72
ambulances 88, 206
American Heart Assoc. 199, 214
aminoacids 121, 139
aminophylline 53, 116
amiodarone 111
analgesic 44, 114
Anectine (succinylcholine) 116
anemia 144
anesthesiologist 187, 191, 204, 207
anesthesia 65
angina 129
angiography 141
ante-flexion 182
anticonvulsants 145
antihistamine 213

anuria 92
aortic aneurysm 91, 176
apallic syndrome 149
Apgar's scoring system 164
Aramine (metaraminol) 106, 168
Armed Forces 210
arrest time 149, 160
arrhythmia manikin 192
arterial catheter 95, 100
arterial PO_2, O_2 content, O_2 transport 73, 75, 141, 142
arterial PO_2, pH 53, 73, 141, 142
arterial pressure 142
artificial ventilation 57, 181
asphyxia 45, 76, 123, 165, 167
aspiration 25, 35, 53, 59, 66, 92, 115, 138, 177
aspirator (suction) 165
assisted ventilation 56, 57, 74
asthma 53, 112, 115, 181
astride position 86
asystole 76, 102, 104, 121, 123, 170, 176
atherosclerosis 181
ATP 148
atrioventricular block 126
atropine 98, 112, 115, 125, 129, 168, 173
audiotape 189, 192
augmentation of blood flow (CPR) 84
Australia 189
automatic defibrillation 136
autoregulation of CBF 148
autotransfusion 90, 92

Backboard 86
back blows 25, 27, 28, 164
back-pressure arm-lift artif. vent 56
backward tilt of head 10, 16, 18, 20, 181
bag-valve-mask-oxygen 62, 64, 66, 82, 166
Baltimore 189
banked blood 120, 176
barbiturate 116, 145, 148, 178
base deficit/excess 109, 110
basic life support 11, 14, 184, 192, 199
beclomethasone 53
bellows-mask unit 15
beta receptors, blockers 103, 112, 131
bicarbonate 167, 168, 173, 176, 178

bigeminal rhythm (EKG) 125
biological death 148
Bird Mark VII ventilator 68
bleeding 88, 92
blind defibrillation 169
blind intubation 45
blood infusion 118, 119, 120
blood gases 67, 100, 102, 167
blood sugar 141
blood viscosity 147
blood volume 92, 110, 111, 116, 176
bone marrow emboli 182
bradycardia 85, 112, 126, 171
brain damage 10, 76, 137, 146, 147
brain death 148, 154, 156, 158
brain-oriented life support 140, 142
brain resuscitation 10, 144, 147
breaking the victim 177
breathing support 11, 56, 88
bretylium (Bretylol) 104, 112
bronchitis, bronchospasm 16, 53, 65, 116
bronchoscopy 36, 46, 53
Brook airway 62
burns 161, 180
bystanders 207

C-A-B sequence 87, 169
calcium, Ca blockers 106, 107, 115, 148, 168
calories 151
campaigns, public 186
carbohydrates 121
cardiac arrest 87, 150, 172
cardiac death 153
cardiac output 79
cardiac tamponade 88, 140, 174
Cardiazol 168
cardiogenic (pump) failure (shock) 108, 140
cardiologist 204
cardiopulmonary-cerebral resuscitation
    (CPCR) 10, 13, 14, 216
cardioscope 133
cardiovascular collapse 121
cardiovascular support 138, 139
cardioversion 125, 131
carotid sinus 126
categorization of hospitals 210
catheter inside and outside needles 95
cats (practice) 193
CAT scanning 141
central venous route, press. (CVP), blood
    95, 98, 139, 144
cerebral edema 115, 116, 138, 146
cerebral electric impedance 144
cerebral performance categories (CPC) 151

cerebral perfusion (CBF), oxygenation 79,
    84, 148, 154
cerebral resuscitation 15, 137, 148, 209
cerebral trauma 137, 147
certification in CPR 198, 214
cervical collar 213
checklists (skill tests) 198-203
chest injury 12
chest-pressure arm-lift artif. vent. 10, 56
chest thrusts 26, 27, 164
chest thumper 86
chest tube 54
children 10, 28, 37, 46, 59, 60, 77, 161
chin support 18
chlorpromazine 116
choke saver 25
choking 23, 25
circulation (depression, support) 10, 11, 57,
    74-76, 211
civic auditorium 211
clearing pharynx 24, 29, 47
Cleveland 191
clofilium 111, 112
closed chest CPR 77, 91
clotting deficiency 119
Club of Mainz 210, 216
coagulation 120
Cole endotracheal tube 46, 168
colloid osmotic pressure 74, 99, 117, 139
colloids 116, 119, 174
coma 19, 33, 45, 47, 87, 142, 149, 152, 181,
    209
combinations of IPPV and ECC 81
committees 11, 204
communications (center) 206
community-wide organization (EMS) 206
compliance 75
complications 186
complications of tracheal intubation 47
compression/relaxation time ratio 84
conscious patient 35, 45
continuous positive airway pressure (CPAP)
    57, 71
continuous positive pressure ventilation
    (CPPV) 21, 53, 57
controlled ventilation (CV) 56, 57, 73
control of hemorrhage 87
convulsions 60, 111
coordinators 192
Coramine 168
coronary care units 210
coronary ischemia 131, 178
cortical death 160
corticosteroids 115, 141, 142

cost-effectiveness 26
cough-CPR 169
countershock 94, 102, 111, 125, 133, 135, 169, 174
CPCR services 204, 206
CPD blood preservation 120
CPK (CSF) 144
CPR basic life support 198, 212
CPR machines 86
CPR outside hospital 85
CPR services 210
CPR time 149
craniotomy 88
crash cart 205
crash intubation 193
cricothyrotomy 25, 49, 51
criteria for passing 198
critical care medicine 148, 207
critical care triage 156
crossed-finger maneuver 24
croup 162
crowd control 211
crushing chest injury 181
CSF drainage 143
CSF pH 144, 148
cuff (endotracheal) 37, 40, 41
cut-down 95
curricula (courses) 188
cyanosis 76, 166
cyclic AMP 144
cylinder (O_2) 71
Czechoslovakia 208

Death (certification) 148, 154, 160, 178
defibrillation 10, 85, 103, 112, 131, 132, 135, 162, 173, 180, 188, 191
definitions 217
delivery 165
Demerol (meperidine) 44, 114, 116
dentist 188
designated team response 205
developing countries 216
dexamethasone 53, 115, 116
dextrans 118, 119
dextrose 116, 143
dialysis 74
diarrhea 121
diazepam (Valium) 116, 140, 142
digitalis (digoxin) 112, 125, 126
diphenylhydantoin (Dilantin, phenytoin) 125, 140, 142, 146, 147
direct current (DC) countershock 131, 132
disaster medicine 210
disseminated intravasc. coagulation (DIC) 138

distress signal (choking) 25
distributive shock 140
diuretic 74, 113, 114, 117, 141, 143
diving 75, 177
dobutamine 108
dofilium 112
dog laboratory 191
dopamine 107, 108, 115, 179
"do not resuscitate" 153
driver's license, driving 187, 211
drowning 131, 147, 161, 177
drugs (and fluids) 11, 92, 94, 102, 142, 168, 188, 191, 213
dysrhythmias 111, 123, 124, 147, 179

Education 183, 207
EKG telemetry 208
elastic bandage 88
Elder valve 67
electric countershock (defibrillation) 131, 133, 135
electric shock (pole top) 76, 131, 180
electrocardiogram (EKG) 121, 122, 126, 134, 154, 170, 176, 179
electrocardiographic (EKG) diagnosis 11, 94, 121, 124, 191
electroencephalogram (EEG) 76, 143, 144, 149, 154
electrolytes 74, 116, 119, 139, 141
electromechanical dissociation 102, 121, 123, 173
elevation of bleeding site 87, 89
emergency airway control 17
emergency artificial ventilation 56
emergency care (medicine, department, physician) 33, 88, 92, 206, 207, 210
emergency medical services (EMS) 11, 168, 208, 209
emphysema 57, 173
empirical countershock 136
emergency med. technician (EMT) 207
encephalitis 148
endotracheal intubation 10, 35, 38, 44, 47, 84, 164, 166, 182, 193
enzymes 144
epiglottitis 53, 162
epinephrine (Adrenaline) 53, 87, 94, 104, 115, 134, 167, 168, 173, 176
epistaxis 44
equipment 192, 199, 211, 212
esophageal electrode 136
esophageal gastric tube airway 33
esophageal obturator airway 32
esophageal stethoscope 41, 121

ethacrynic acid 114, 116, 179
ethics 157
etomidate 140, 142
euthanasia 160
evaluation 92, 137, 148, 207
evolution 216
exhaled air ventilation 20, 58, 61
expiratory (naso-pharyngeal) obstruction 60
external cardiac compression 10, 77, 78, 162
external hemorrhage 87, 88
extra-cellular fluid 117
extra-cerebral (life support) 137, 140, 142
exsanguinating hemorrage 91, 123, 131, 174
extrication 91, 210
extubation 46

Failure of ventilation and oxygenation 74
fat embolism 140
feedback 190, 204
femoral artery catheterization 76, 100, 101
fentanyl 114
fetus 168
fiberoptic (flexible) bronchoscope 53
fiberoptic laryngoscope 46
fibrillation patterns and treatment 11, 94, 128
films, training 190
finger behind teeth maneuver 24
finger sweep 27
FIO$_2$ 74, 118, 139
fireman 184, 188, 211
first aid (kit) 183, 196
first responders 188
fist pacing 129, 170
fixed pupils 154
flail chest 138
flow meter 71
fluid resuscitation 12, 74, 91, 92, 116, 142
fluorocarbons (Fluosol DA) 120, 121
Flunarizine 107
folding mask (Laerdal) 62, 63
foreign body obstruction 25, 161
forward displacement of mandible 16
furosemide 114

Gastric intubation 48
gauging (triage) 11, 137, 149
gelatine 118, 119
general response (CPR team) 204
Germany 208
Glasgow Coma Scale 149
Glasgow Outcome Categories 151
global ischemia 138, 142, 150
globulin 119
glucocorticoid 141

glucose 117, 148
glycerol 141
Good Samaritan Act 214
GOT (enzyme) 144
guidelines 183, 187

Halothane 148
handkerchief 60
head injury 146, 181
head-tilt 12, 21, 161
health care personnel 188
heart associations 186
heart attack (disease, failure) 76, 129, 145, 209
heart block 123, 126, 129, 170
"hearts too good to die" (Beck) 178
heat stroke 180
helicopters 209, 210
hematocrit 73, 117, 118, 139, 141, 142
hemodilution 118, 145, 147
hemoglobin 73, 75, 110, 176
hemolytic reactions 118
hemorrhage 89, 90, 105, 119, 144, 172, 174, 190
hemothorax 88, 182
heparinization, heparin 100, 145, 147
hepatitis 118
high frequency IPPV, ventilator, oscillation 50, 69
high altitude 75
history 10
hospital wide resuscitation (team) 191, 205
hospitals 204, 209-212
how to teach 194
human corpses 191, 194
human mentation 11
human volunteers 190
humanizing 137
humidification 70, 71
hydroxyethyl starch 120
hyperbaric O$_2$ 75
hyper (hypo) carbia 17, 46, 137
hypernatremia 108, 167
hypertension 113, 137, 140, 142, 145, 147, 179
hyperthermia 180
hyperventilation 72, 108, 140, 178
hypoglycemia 144, 165
hypopharyngeal obstruction 18, 32
hypotension 57, 137, 167, 179
hypothermia 119, 141, 143-147, 165, 173, 178, 180
hypovolemia (shock) 90, 105, 117, 140, 145
hypoxemia 17, 46, 76, 137
hypoxia time 149

ICP monitoring 140, 143, 146, 147, 148
immobilization 142, 145, 146
impedance (cerebral) 133,
Inderal (propranolol) 112
infant resuscitation 28, 46, 60, 62, 77, 81 161
infection 144, 147
informed consent 215
injurious performance 189
instructors-coordinators 189, 198
insulin 148
insult time 149
intake and output 139
intensive care (therapy) units (ICU) 10, 11,
    69, 72, 137, 204, 206
IPPV, IPPB, IMV 10, 21, 53, 56-58, 62,
    68, 74, 84, 139, 174, 177
internal hemorrhage 88, 90
interposed ventilation (CPR) 84
interstitial emphysema 53
intra-aortic balloon pumping 179
intra-arterial infusion 176
intracardiac injection 97
intracranial pressure (ICP) 140, 141, 143
intramuscular route (drugs) 98
intrathoracic hemorrhage 181
intrathoracic pressure 79, 91, 172
intratracheal medication 95, 104
intravenous infusions 84, 87, 94, 97, 116,
    139, 174
intubating awake 44, 191
intubation manikins 3, 19, 191, 196
iron lung 69
irreversible shock 140
ischemic brain edema 144
ischemic heart disease 10
isoelectric EEG 157
isoproterenol (Isuprel) 105, 106, 108, 115,
    125, 129, 168, 179

Jaw thrust 10, 18, 19, 21, 22, 62, 181, 191
jet ventilation 69
jugular vein catheter 94
joules (watt seconds) 131, 132

Knowledge 183, 189, 196, 198
Kreiselman bellows 64

Labor 167
laboratory   (animals)   191,   194,   212
lactate 144
lanatoside 113
Laerdal RFB II resusci-folding bag 65, 66
Laerdal's manikins 196
Laerdal's self-training system 192
Laerdal pocket mask 62

laparotomy 88, 91, 176
larynx, laryngospasm 16, 22, 42, 177
laryngoscopy (view) 37, 39, 40, 42, 46, 134,
    168, 173, 179
laryngectomee 60
laryngotracheobronchitis 53
lasix 114
law 144, 157, 214
lay public 184, 186, 206
LDH (enzyme) 144
lenient passing criteria 198
letting die 160
Levophed (norepinephrine) 105, 168
lidocaine (Xylocaine) 45, 98, 102, 110, 111,
    115, 125, 131, 168
lightning 131
life support 137, 183, 186
life support units (stations) 208, 212
life supporting first aid 12, 87, 91, 183, 192,
    196, 198
lifeguard 184, 188, 211
liver injury 80, 91, 182
living will 214
lung rupture 57, 65

Magill's forceps 45
manuals (see teaching)
manikins 190, 192, 194
mannitol 116, 141, 143
masks 61, 65, 71, 193
mass training 186
manual O_2 ventilators 67
measures of CPCR steps 13, 184, 194
mediastinal shift 53
Medic alert 92
metabolism 74, 148
mechanical ventilation 44
mentation 137
medical director 187, 208
medical practice act 214
medical students 184
microcirculation 119, 140, 148
military anti-shock trousers (MAST) 84, 88,
    90
metaproterenol 53, 116
metaraminol (Aramine) 104, 106, 115, 168
methoxarmine 126
meperidine (Demerol) 44, 114, 116
methylprednisolone 53, 115, 116
Mobitz I, II A-V block 126
monitoring 85, 168
monkeys 193
morphine 114, 116, 180
mouth piece 71
mouth-to-adjunct (mask, airway) 31, 61, 62,
    82

mouth-to-mouth 10, 20, 22, 58, 61, 87, 177, 180, 181, 186, 189
mouth-to-mouth-nose (infants) 163
mouth-to-nose 20, 58, 60, 61, 177
mouth-to-trach tube (infants) 166
multi-trauma, multi-organ failure 12, 138, 140, 181
muscle relaxant 41
myocardial ischemia, failure, infarction 76, 112, 113, 123, 178, 210

Narcan (naloxone) 116, 168
nasogastric tube 48, 59
nasopharyngeal oxygen 72
nasopharyngeal tube 30
nasotracheal tube 35, 44
nasotracheal suctioning 30
near-drowning 53, 66, 177
nebulizer 65, 70
neck injury 177
necklift 18, 161
nembutal (pentobarbital) 140
neonate (newborn) 163, 164, 168, 169
neosynephrine (phenylephrine) 104
neurologic deficit 138
"new" CPR 84
news media 187
nitroglycerin nitroprusside 113, 115, 179, 180
non-physician personnel 188, 214
non-rebreathing valve 64
norepinephrine 104, 105, 115, 168, 179
normal values 217
Normosol 119
Norway 189
novacaine (procaine) 111
nurse 184, 188, 204

Obesity 28
obstetrics 164, 169
obstructive shock 140
oculocephalic, oculovestibular reflex 151
office building 211
open-chest (cardiac) resuscitation 10, 11, 87, 98, 172, 181
operating room (suite) 207, 212
organizations, organizers 192, 204, 207
oral fluids 121
oronasal masks 72
oropharyngeal tube 31
orotracheal intubation 35, 39, 43
osmolality, osmotic pressure 74, 108, 117, 139, 141, 142
osmotherapy 141, 144-147
overall performance category (OPC) 151

Oxford bellows 64
oxygen 41, 62, 64, 68, 85, 166, 177, 178, 211
oxygenation 49, 56, 72, 74
oxygen concentration, (inhaled), toxicity 70, 73
oxygen delivery systems 70, 72
oxygen mask, nipple 62, 63
oxygen, 100% test 75
oxygen powered ventilator 68
oxygen transport 118

Pacing, pacemaker 11, 85, 129, 183
packed red blood cells 120
$PaCO_2$ 74, 100, 109
pancuronium (Pavulon) 116, 140
panorganic death 148
paralysis 182
paramedics 33, 207, 211
parasympatholytic 112
passing criteria (teaching-testing) 198, 199
PEEP 21, 57, 66-68, 74, 75, 139, 167, 177
pentobarbital (nembutal) 116, 140, 143, 146
pentothal (thiopental) 116, 140, 143-146
pethidine (meperidine, Demerol) 45, 114, 116
pH 73, 100, 102, 108-110
phases of CPCR 11, 13, 16, 184, 194
phenytoin (Dilantin) 140, 146, 147
pheochromocytoma 112
philosophy 216
phlebotomy 114, 180
pharyngeal intubation 30, 64
pharyngeal suction 29
phenylephrine (neosynephrine) 45
physicians 184, 188, 207-209
picrotoxin 168
pitfalls of CPR 181
Pittsburgh 147, 189, 198, 201, 202, 203
Pittsburgh-Glasgow Coma Scale 149
Pittsburgh-Glasgow Performance Categories 151
plasma infusion 120
plasma volume 117, 142
plasma substitutes 174, 176
pleural drainage, pneumothorax 53, 54, 88, 181, 182
pneumonia 76
pneumoperitoneum 53
PO_2 (PO_2 gradient) 75, 100, 118, 180
pocket mask 63
poikilothermia (hypothermia) 147
poisoning 161
poletop resuscitation 86
police 184, 188, 211

positioning 19, 87, 91
positive negative pressure ventilation (PNPV) 56, 57
positive pressure (ventilation) 21, 56, 57, 75
post-anoxic (ischemic) brain damage 144, 178
potassium (depletion) 113, 119, 131, 143
precordial thump 170
pregnancy 28, 169
pre-hospital advanced life support 208, 209
premature ventricular (PVC) and atrial (PAC) contractions 110, 125
pressure bandage 87, 89
primary cardiac arrest 76
primary, secundary survey 92
procaine, procaine amide 111, 125, 179
progressive pulmonary consolidation 138
prolonged life support 11, 15, 185, 193, 195
pronestyl (procaine amide) 111
propranolol (Inderal) 112, 125
protection, cerebral 134
protocols, resuscitation 204, 208
public 187, 210
pulmonary artery catheterization, 99, 113, 118, 139, 179
pulmonary edema and congestion 44, 65, 76, 113, 114, 138, 180
pulmonary embolism 140, 173
pulselessness 74, 121, 128, 162, 209
pupillary dilatation 76, 77, 85
push-pull methods of artif. vent. 56

Quality of life 151
quinidine 112, 125, 131

Radial artery cath. 100
radio, telephone (EMS) 206-208
rapid intubation 41
red blood cell infusion 116, 120
Red Cross 186
recording manikin 190
record keeping 205
recovery room 212
reducing valve 71
regional hospitals 209, 211
regurgitation 21, 35, 44, 59, 80
renal failure (ischemia) 74, 91, 137
reperfusion promotion 137, 144
"rescue pull" 87, 91, 93
research 207
res ipsa loquitur 214
respiratory distress 10, 138, 139, 165, 209
respiratory therapist 205
resuscitation (teams) 183, 204, 210
Resuscitation Research Center (RRC) 201, 202

resuscitators 68, 144
retraining, retesting 188, 189
rib fractures 80, 182
Ringer's solution 117, 119, 121, 167, 174
Riva-Rocci (blood pressure) 121
Robertshaw valve 67
R-on-T PVCs (EKG) 126

Saline infusion 117, 119
salvageability 154
scene, spot (EMS) 207
school children 187
sea water drowning 177
secondary cardiac arrest 76
seizures (convulsions) 60, 140, 143
self-help 169
self-refilling bag-valve mask 64
self-training systems 189, 192, 196
sepsis, septic shock 137, 140
serial defibrillation 134
sequence of CPR steps 60, 81
shock 76, 87, 91-93, 116, 118, 121, 138, 140, 165, 167, 179, 210
shunting (pulmonary) 66, 73, 117
Siggaard Andersen nomogram 109
sitting position 180
skill practice 183, 189, 190, 198
skill tests (on manikins, etc.) 198, 200-203
skull screw (ICP) monitoring 141, 143
slides (teaching) 190
"social death" (vegetative state) 149
sodium bicarbonate 91, 94, 102, 108, 115, 167
sodium chloride infusion 116
Soviet Union 208
speaking tracheostomy tube 51
spinal cord injury 177, 182
spine board, splints 213
spontaneous breathing (SB) with continuous positive airway pressure (CPAP) 56, 58, 66, 74
sputum examination 139
stabilization of patient 182, 211
stable side position 19, 92
staffing of CPR services 210
standards of CPCR 204, 208
starch solutions IV 118, 119
status asthmaticus 53, 106
steps of CPCR 11, 13, 184, 194
sternal compressions 78, 83
steroids 53
Stokes-Adams syndrome 106, 129
stomach 21, 32, 41, 181
suction 29, 41, 166

sudden cardiac death 10, 87, 169, 178
suffocation 161
surgeon 88, 204, 207
supported supine aligned position 19, 92
surveillance of patients 211
suxamethonium (succinylcholine) 116
Swan-Ganz pulmonary artery catheter 99
sweeping the pharynx 24
switching CPR between operators 85
sympathomimetic amines 103, 104
synchronization of CPR 135

Tachydysrhythmias 126, 129, 179
tank ventilator (iron lung) 69
target groups for teaching 187
teaching methods 11, 183, 184, 188, 189,
    192, 196, 198, 214
team response 86, 205, 207, 215
telemetry (EKG) 123
telephone number (EMS) 205, 206
tension pneumothorax 53
termination of resuscitation 153, 155, 214
testing of trainees, test results 189, 198
THAM (tris buffer) 110
thiopental (pentothal) 116, 140, 143, 145-
    147
thoracotomy 88, 91, 175, 183
throat-E-vac 25
thrusts, abdominal and chest 25, 164
thumb-jaw-lift maneuver 22, 23
thump (chest thump) 171
"thumpers" (CPR machines) 86
thyrotoxicosis 112
tissue oxygenation and perfusion 75
titration of therapy 215
tongue jaw-lift maneuver 24
tonsil suction tip 29
topical anesthesia 44, 45
tourniquet 88, 89
tracheobronchial suction 29
tracheotomy 29, 36, 51, 52, 60, 181
transportation 86, 183, 207
transfusion 117
translaryngeal jet insufflation 25, 50, 69
trauma 10, 12, 19, 60, 92, 121, 144, 161
triage 137, 148, 155
trigeminal rhythm 125
triple airway maneuver 16, 21, 23, 63
T-tube for oxygen 71
two-hands jaw-lift maneuver 22
two-operator CPR 83

Umbilical artery 167, 168
unconsciousness 17, 60, 76, 191

universal emerg. tel. number 207
unwitnessed arrest 102, 171

Vacuum (suction) 168
Valsalve maneuver 126, 170
vasoconstriction (dilation) 91, 113, 114, 179
Vasoxyl (methoxamine) 104
vegetative state 149, 152, 156, 160
ventilating bronchoscope 53
ventilation patterns 56, 72, 74, 84, 162, 191
ventilation devices 67
ventricular (CSF, ICP) catheter 141, 143
ventricular extrasystoles 110, 125
ventricular tachycardia and fibrillation 102,
    110, 112, 121-125, 129, 131, 169, 170, 178
Venturi mask 72
venous cannulation 95, 97, 176
venous return 75
Verapamil (Ca antagonist) 107, 111, 126
vitamins 139
voltage (defibrillation) 132
volume set ventilation 68
volunteers 208
vomiting 177

Wall oxygen 70
watt seconds (joules) 131, 152
weaning (controlled ventilation) 75
Wenckebach A-V block 126
World Fed Soc. of Anesth. (WFSA) 198, 216
whai to teach whom 184
World Health Org. (WHO) 216
witnessed arrest 102, 170
wounds 88, 92
written tests 198

Xiphoid process 80, 98
Xylocaine (lidocaine) 45, 102, 110, 168

Yoke 71

238

If you decide to use this form routinely in your hospital, contact P. Safar for participation in CPCR case Registry: RRC, 3434 Fifth Avenue, University of Pittsburgh, Pittsburgh, PA 15260 U.S.A. Telephone: (412) 624-6735.

CASE REPORT FORM
Cardiopulmonary-Cerebral Resuscitation Attempt
(suggested by P. Safar, WFSA-CPR Committee)
Complete one form for each patient.
Insert data or check what is applicable.

Reporting physician, name ....

phone number ....

Hospital, name ....

address (incl. city, country) ....

Patient, name ....

hospital number ....

Age (years) ....

Male ☐   Female ☐

Date of arrest   month ☐☐ , day ☐☐ , year ☐☐☐☐

Location of arrest: outside hospital ☐   in hospital: Operating room ☐
Emergency Department ☐
ICU-CCU ☐
Other location ☐

IMMEDIATELY PRE-ARREST
No background disease, healthy ☐

With background disease   ☐
if yes, state disease ....

ARREST
Cause of arrest ....

Estimated duration of insult	min : sec
Cardiac arrest (no pulse) without CPR	:
Arrest with CPR-ABC	:
Severe hypotension or hypoxemia without CPR-ABC	:

Continued on next page

RESUSCITATION (check all applicable)

Mouth-to-mouth/nose	☐	Electric countershock	☐
Other IPPV method	☐	Drugs during CPR-ABC	☐
Tracheal intubation	☐	Successful restoration of	
Ext. cardiac compression	☐	spontaneous circulation yes	☐
Open-chest cardiac massage	☐	no	☐
EKG taken during arrest	☐		
if yes — VF	☐	if yes, was patient	
asystole	☐	admitted to ICU? yes	☐
QRS complexes	☐	no	☐

POST-ARREST (follow for at least 4 weeks or until earlier death)
Patient followed over .... days/weeks/months/years (check)
Recovered consciousness: yes ☐ no ☐
  if yes, ... min/hours/days after restoration of spontaneous circulation
Discharged from hospital .... days post-arrest
  discharged alive ☐ dead ☐
If discharged alive, is still alive .... days/weeks/months/years post-arrest
  died after discharge .... days/weeks/months/years post-arrest
If died, cause of death ....

PERFORMANCE CAPABILITY (check one for each time)

	Pre-arrest	Best while in hospital	At time of discharge from hospital	Best after discharge from hospital
1) Normal	☐	☐	☐	☐
2) Conscious, moderately disabled because of:				
a) Brain dysfunction;	☐	☐	☐	☐
b) Other organ system dysfunction	☐	☐	☐	☐
3) Conscious, severely disabled because of:				
a) Brain dysfunction;	☐	☐	☐	☐
b) Other organ system dysfunction	☐	☐	☐	☐
4) Unconscious (not brain death),vegetative ☐		☐	☐	☐
5) Brain death, death	☐	☐	☐	☐
6) Under anesthesia	☐	☐	☐	☐

Comments: